the

(FIT)

FORMULA

The World's Leading Experts Reveal
Proven Strategies for Optimal Health,
Fitness, and Nutrition

—— FEATURING ——
THE WORLD FITNESS ELITE

Published by CelebrityPress™, Orlando, FL
A division of The Celebrity Branding Agency®

Celebrity Branding® is a registered trademark
Printed in the United States of America.

ISBN: 9780983340492
LCCN: 2011936939

This publication is designed to provide accurate and authoritative
information with regard to the subject matter covered. It is sold with
the understanding that the publisher is not engaged in rendering legal,
accounting, or other professional advice. If legal advice or other expert
assistance is required, the services of a competent professional should
be sought. The opinions expressed by the authors in this book are not
endorsed by CelebrityPress™ and are the sole responsibility of the
author rendering the opinion.

Most CelebrityPress™ titles are available at special quantity discounts
for bulk purchases for sales promotions, premiums, fundraising, and
educational use. Special versions or book excerpts can also be created
to fit specific needs.

For more information, please write:

CelebrityPress™,
520 N. Orlando Ave, #2
Winter Park, FL 32789

or call 1.877.261.4930

Visit us online at www.CelebrityPressPublishing.com

the
(FIT)
FORMULA

Table of Contents

Foreword
By Dax Moy 13

Chapter 1
Eating for YOUR Body Type
By Tyler English 17

Chapter 2
Eat More and Stop Exercising—
A 21st Century Approach to Health and Fitness
By John O'Connell 29

Chapter 3
**Why Women Store Fat In The Lower
Body And What To Do**
By Paul Mort 39

Chapter 4
**Putting Weight Loss Theory into Practice and
Maintaining the Results in a Balanced Way**
By Tim Saye – London 43

Chapter 5

Are your Hormones Making You Fat?

By Graham Webb & Steve Butters 51

Chapter 6

The Simplest Most Effective Nutrition Plan

By Trevor Buccieri 63

Chapter 7

Fitness and Weight Loss for Baby Boomer Women

By Becky Williamson 73

Chapter 8

How to Develop Hero Focus

By Oliver Chapman 81

Chapter 9

Be Fit For Life

By Damien Maher 89

Chapter 10

Goal Setting, Action Planning, and Achievement

By Nick Berry 105

Chapter 11

Get Off The Scale To Get Results

By Holly Rigsby 113

Chapter 12

Kaizen Fitness and the Hedgehog Concept: A Model for Long Term Fitness Planning

By Timothy J. Ward 121

Chapter 13

The First Step to Fitness Success

By Pat Rigsby 129

Chapter 14

The Power of Intention

By Dean Coulson 135

Chapter 15

Your Personal Trainer Isn't So S.M.A.R.T.

By Mike Bach 143

Chapter 16

The Fit Formula –
Because You're Worth It...

By Sam Feltham 153

Chapter 17

The Fit Formula –
Your Journey of a Lifetime

By Nicky Sehgal 161

Chapter 18
Inside the Mindset of an Athlete
By Brad Hall 169

Chapter 19
Realism For Fitness
By Dustin Williams 177

Chapter 20
**Igniting Shift To Solutions:
30 Minutes For 30 Days!**
By Ron Jones 185

Chapter 21
**The Complete 30-Minute
Training Session –**
Feel Better, Get Stronger, and Look
Like You've Always Wanted To
By Luka Hocevar 193

Chapter 22
**Metabolic Resistance Training:
The Fat Loss Formula**
By Clint Howard, MS 201

Chapter 23
Core Concepts For Sexy Abs
By Ryan Riley, CSCS 209

Chapter 24
Unstable Surface Training Myths
By Tony Larkin 217

Chapter 25
Train Smarter Not Harder
By Steve Long 225

Chapter 26
From Joe To Pro -
Without Machines
By Kyle Jakobe 233

Chapter 27
**How To Design 'Guaranteed Results'
Training Programs**
By Jon Le Tocq 241

Chapter 28
Self-Limiting Exercises
By Alwyn and Rachel Cosgrove 251

Foreword

By Dax Moy

With so many books on fitness and fat-loss already in print, it may seem to some that pretty well anything that can be said about the subject has been said already. Following that line of reasoning, the addition of yet another book adds little, if anything, to the 'big picture' of achieving lifelong fitness.

Most of the time, those raising such a point would be right. After all, most of the fitness and fat-loss information that finds its way onto our bookshelves is often little more than a very general rehash of ideas that are decades old. (Sometimes more!) They do little to enhance our ability to get to where we want to go faster, and stay there longer, than we already do.

And if that's not happening, then, at least to my way of thinking, these kinds of books are nothing more than 'padding', that superfluous 'extra' that adds nothing but even more information to sift through… as if we didn't have enough already!

This is one of the reasons why, in just over a decade within the health and fitness profession, and with a pretty high standing among my peers, I've not gone out of my way to recommend more than a handful of fitness or fat-loss related books. I simply didn't want to be seen to be adding to all of the 'noise' that's already in circulation around this topic.

The way I see it, most people are already drowning in fitness and fat-loss information. Information that they're not sure how to use – whilst at the same time thirsting for the knowledge that'll truly make the difference in their pursuit of their goals.

So when I was asked to write the foreword to this book, I set some pretty simple and straightforward criteria in place to see whether or not I'd be happy to recommend it to others.

The first question I asked myself was, "Does this add anything new that people didn't know before?" That, of course, is a difficult question to answer when you think about it. After all, I have no way of knowing exactly how well-read you or anyone else reading this book is already, right?

That said, I'm fairly certain that new and intermediate exercisers will learn a lot of valuable information that'll take them closer to their goals. In addition, the even more advanced exercisers will be exposed to new applications of older ideas that they're already familiar with.

So far so good I guess, but remember, I said that simply providing information in and of itself just wasn't enough for me to feel comfortable promoting this or any other book. For that to happen, it would have to take over where information left off. It would have to provide meaningful knowledge.

So the second question I asked myself was, "Is what's being shared here coming from those who've had consistently predictable and reproducible results?" It wasn't enough that the information sounded plausible, I wanted to know if the contributors had a track record of getting great results for their clients again and again by using the concepts they'd shared in the book. After all, the surest signs of mastery are predictability and reproducibility, right? ANYONE can get a couple of 'one-off' success stories under their belts, but it takes a real master to do it over and over.

Thankfully, as I worked my way through the contributors, one thing became crystal clear; each of them had been consistently helping their clients to get their results faster and keep them longer than fully 99% of the industry – and had 'sackloads of evidence' to prove it.

Seriously, this book The FIT Formula, has some of the best fitness professionals in the business contributing to it, both those who are already world-renowned for their approaches as well as those whose names may not be on your radar right now, but who are undoubtedly set to be the fitness superstars of the future.

Don't waste this opportunity to use this wealth of knowledge!

Grab it with both hands. Apply what you learn from the following pages, and whatever health and fitness goals you're currently working toward will be achieved far faster and last longer than they would otherwise. I guarantee it.

Within these pages lie all the education and the motivation you'll ever need to get to where you want to go. All that's missing, in order for you to actually get there, is the magic ingredient that only you can provide… the perspiration, or at least, the dedication to apply what you learn.

Add that and big things are on their way, I promise.

To your success!

Dax Moy

The UK's Leading Personal Trainer, Founder Of Personal Trainer Success Academy
Author of the best-selling *MAGIC Hundred Goal Achievement Program*, *The Look Great Naked Challenge* and *The Elimination Diet Detox Plan*.

CHAPTER 1

Eating for YOUR Body Type

By Tyler English

A single search of the word "diet" into Google will leave you with 565 million results in about 0.16 seconds.

Now imagine if you could actually transform your body that fast. Though as you've probably figured out by now, it takes a little more work than that. I'm not here to tell you the impossible, but what I can tell you, is that aside from the thousands of diet plans out there – YOU ARE IN CONTROL!

Yes, there is something that you can do to help lose body fat, gain lean muscle and feel better. It will take a little bit of work, and it is not a miracle fix. I hope that after reading this chapter you will understand how my experiences, both personal and professional, have allowed me to help transform the way I "diet" – as well as the approach my clients take when dieting.

This is a way for you to discover how you are unique, how you are in control of your body and how you can help transform that same body into the best shape of your life.

The Skinny Athlete

My goals when I first started exercising in my teen years were not to lose body fat, but to gain weight. I know, hardly what most of you want to hear. Being an athletic skinny kid growing up I found it hard to put on weight. The end result, I would get overpowered by bigger kids on the soccer field, basketball court and I never was the "homerun champ" in Little League. I actually made every All-Star team without ever hitting a homerun, well unless I count those 2 inside-the-park homeruns.

At that age I ate what ever I wanted but would always maintain an athletic skinny frame. This was likely because I played every sport imaginable and my caloric output most likely superseded my caloric input.

I grew up with an Italian grandfather so for me it was always, eat more food, and to grow, eat more food. When your grandfather's nickname was "Bull" you listened. I didn't see the healthy side of food until I was in college. By then I had put on a good amount of muscle in the later years of high school through strength training and eating more, so for me, it was easier to make the smarter choice.

Don't get me wrong, I most definitely was still the typical college kid, I just made time to workout and chose better meal options.

To me, putting on muscle always had meant, "eat protein." After all, that is what all the popular magazines were telling me to do.

I first discovered my body type when I was in college but I never really grasped the concept of eating for my body type until I began my transition into the natural bodybuilder world. It was here that I learned why my body could consume more carbohydrates then most people.

Genetically You ARE Different

The number of genetic fat cells we possess can be significantly different from person to person. The end result is it makes it harder for some to lose weight. I can tell you from experience that only in a small percentage of people do genetics play a major role in making it easier to gain weight.

When I first tell someone this they immediately look to blame their genetics and I'm not going to downplay the role of your metabolism. It is important and plays a large role in the success of weight management.

The keys to success actually have a lot to do with WHAT you eat and in WHAT amounts.

Have you ever heard the term "eating for your body type"?

Your body will typically fall into one of three body types or somato-types: ectomorph, mesomorph, and endomorph. It's very uncommon for a person to fit perfectly into just one of the three categories. Many times a person's lifestyle can alter what may have been their natural body type. In this case, an almost hybrid body type is created.

So What Body Type Are You?

First we you need to look at the different somatotype or body types:

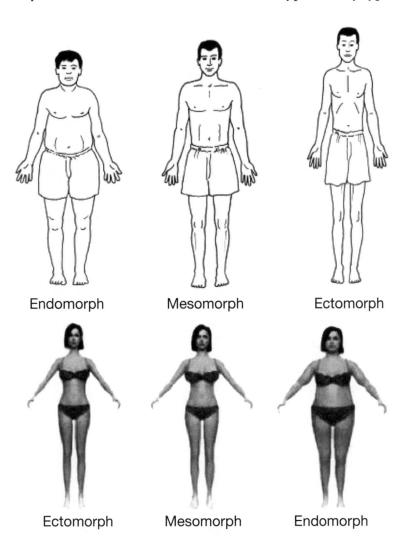

Endomorph	Mesomorph	Ectomorph

Ectomorph	Mesomorph	Endomorph

Ectomorph

An ectomorphic somatotype is naturally thin with skinny limbs with stringy muscles. Think of a person whose body type resembles that of an endurance athlete. These are the people whose body is thyroid dominant – meaning they have a fast metabolism and a higher carbohydrate tolerance. Growing up I found myself in this category but knew nothing about it. For me, it would have been easier to eat more carbohydrates, but instead I found myself consuming all things protein.

Ectomorph Characteristics:
• Small frame and bone structure
• Thin
• Long and stringy muscles
• Flat chest
• Thin shoulders with little width
• Hard to gain weight
• Fast metabolism

Usually ectomorphs find it very difficult to gain weight due to their fast metabolism. Ectomorphs can usually lose body fat easily with small changes to diet though making it extra difficult to hold onto valuable lean muscle mass.

Mesomorph

A mesomorphic somatotype carries a more naturally muscular or athletic frame. This body type finds it easier to build muscle as they tend to be testosterone and growth hormone dominant – meaning they have a easier time holding onto lean muscle gains although they gain fat more easily than ectomorphs.

Mesomorph Characteristics:
• Naturally muscular
• Athletic
• Strong
• Well-defined muscles
• Rectangular shaped physique
• Gain muscle easily
• Gain body fat easier than ectomorphs

The mesomorph body type is a great platform for building a lean muscular physique as they find it easier to gain and lose weight. Most mesomorph physiques have larger muscles and naturally muscular physique that can resemble a physique competitor or bodybuilder.

Endomorph

An endomorphic somatotype is naturally broad and thick. The main characteristics are being insulin dominant, having a slow metabolic rate and low carbohydrate tolerance. Their body structure is one of a wider waist, larger bone structure, heavily muscled yet carry extra body fat around the midsection.

Endomorph Characteristics:
• Soft round body
• Shorter build or "stocky"
• Round physique
• Thick arms and legs
• Finds it hard to lose body fat
• Slow metabolism

Due to endomorph's low carbohydrate tolerance and insulin dominant characteristics they often find it very difficult to lose body fat, especially in the central region (abdominal, low back).

A "New" Body Type?

You shouldn't get too hung up on trying to figure out your body type classification. In my experience often times a person's lifestyle can alter what may have been their natural body type, forming almost a hybrid body type. Instead focus on your personal goals.

Take for example my experience as a young athlete. I was more of an ectomorph but have transformed into more of an ecto-mesomorph (athletic and muscular, yet still on the thin side). Or a person who may see their body transform into more of an endo-mesomorph (someone who is heavily muscled and carries extra body fat around the midsection).

This can happen for other reasons as well. I became a hybrid of an ectomorph and mesomorph through my eating and exercise habits yet someone can also be a natural ectomorph who due to years of inactivity and poor food choices might have developed poor insulin sensitivity and carbohydrate tolerance resulting in a mixture of an ecto-mesomorph.

Don't get too hung up on discovering your "exact" body type. For many people it takes proper planning, consistency and time to truly discover what will work for your body and ultimately your body type.

Calories for Your Body Type

I will go out on a limb and say that the majority of the people reading this are looking to lose body fat. Fat loss requires that you achieve a negative energy balance or the result of total calorie expenditure exceeding total calorie intake. What many fail to mention is that whether you track it or not, it still counts. Losing weight and ultimately fat loss is not just about numbers, it's physiology. So remember, your genetics, your body type and your metabolism will play a role in your success. Ultimately, you are still in control as you decide what to consume.

For that same majority, understand these tables are simply calorie estimators and they may vary person to person. The calculations from both contributing factors can be your activity level, current diet and exercise regime.

Fat Loss

For those that have the access to measure body fat percentages the equation is still simple but based on current percentage of body fat and current lean body mass.

Current Body Fat	Calorie Intake
6-12%	17K per pound of LBM
12.1-15%	16K per pound of LBM
15.1-19%	15K per pound of LBM
19.1%-22%	14K per pound of LBM
22.1 or above	13K per pound of LBM

Example A: A woman with the body fat percentage of 22% who weighs 150 pounds would consume 1638 calories.
Step 1: 150 * .22 = 33 (Current bodyweight multiplied by body fat percentage, 22)
Step 2: 150 − 33 = 117 (Current bodyweight minus current pounds of body fat)
Step 3: 117 * 14 = 1638 (Lean Body Mass total multiplied by 14 calories per pound of lean body mass)

Example B: A man with the body fat percentage of 22% who weighs 200 pounds would consume 2184 calories.

Step 1: 200 * .22 = 44 (Current bodyweight multiplied by body fat percentage, 22)

Step 2: 200 − 44 = 156 (Current bodyweight minus current pounds of body fat)

Step 3: 156 * 14 = 2184 (Lean Body Mass total multiplied by 14 calories per pound of lean body mass)

For most people it's difficult to have access to an accurate measurement of body fat. So for these people I've put together a chart to allow you to configure your calorie range needs based entirely on your current bodyweight and activity level.

Activity Level	Weight Loss
Sedentary (minimal exercise)	Bodyweight x 10-12
Moderately Active (3-4 times/wk)	Bodyweight x 12-14
Very Active (5-7 times/wk)	Bodyweight x 14-16

Example A: A sedentary woman weighing 150 pounds who wants to shed body fat would keep her caloric range in between 1500 (150 x 10) and 1800 (150 x 12).

Example B: A moderately active man weighing 225 pounds who wants to shed body fat would keep his caloric range in between 2700 (225 x 12) and 3150 (225 x 14).

Now for those of you out there that are saying "I don't want to lose weight" or "I want to gain weight," I've put together a chart for calorie recommendations as well.

Weight Maintenance

Activity Level	Weight Maintenance
Sedentary	Bodyweight x 12-14
Moderately Active (3-4 times/wk)	Bodyweight x 14-16
Very Active (5-7 times/wk)	Bodyweight x 16-18

Example A: A moderately active woman weighing 140 pounds who wants to maintain her weight would keep her caloric range in between 1960 (140 x 14) and 2240 (140 x 16).

Example B: A moderately active man weighing 180 pounds who wants to maintain his current body weight would keep his caloric range in between 2520 (180 x 14) and 2,880 (180 x 16).

Weight Gain

Activity Level	Weight Loss
Sedentary (minimal exercise)	Bodyweight x 16-18
Moderately Active (3-4 times/ wk)	Bodyweight x 18-20
Very Active (5-7 times/wk)	Bodyweight x 20-22

Example A: A very active female weighing 120 pounds who wants to gain weight would keep her caloric range in between 2,400 (120 x 20) and 2640 (120 x 22).

Example B: A very active male weighing 150 pounds who wants to gain weight would keep his caloric range in between 3,000 (150 x 20) and 3,300 (150 x 22).

Macronutrients For Body Type: The Hidden Secret

As humans, our genetics can play a major role in fat loss. Our body type or somatotype is a way for us to generally categorize our body's structure as well as muscle, fat storage and distribution.

Your body will typically fall into one of three body types:

Ectomorphic: Have lower body fat storage and therefore can consume more carbohydrates, and less protein and less fat.
Recommended Starting Percentages.
Protein: 20 - 25%
Carbohydrates: 55 - 60%
Fat: 20 - 25%

Mesomorphic: Have a stronger ability to control body fat levels. Mesomorphs can consume more protein and fat than that of the ectomorph, yet due to moderate carbohydrate tolerance may need to consume fewer carbohydrates.
Recommended Starting Percentages.
Protein: 30 - 35%

Carbohydrates: 40 - 45%
Fat : 30 % - 35%

Endomorphic: Due to a low tolerance for carbohydrates, endomorphs can succeed with more protein, more fat and less carbohydrates in their daily consumption.

Recommended Starting Percentages.
Protein 35 - 40%
Carbohydrates 25 - 30%
Fat 40 - 45%

Putting It Together

Now that you understand how many calories you need and how your macronutrients will be determined, let's put it all together based on body type, activity level and ultimate goal.

Let's take a 150 pound sedentary client who wants to lose fat.

By taking a look at her I've determined she's an endomorph.

Based on my earlier recommendations her calorie needs will fall between 1500 kcal per day and 1800 kcal per day (bodyweight times 10 to 12)

I've identified her macronutrient ranges to be the following 35% protein, 25% carbohydrates, and 40% fat. (These can always be varied)

So now I need to predetermine the amount of calorie and macronutrient recommendations. To make things easier for her to start, we are going to keep her at 1500 calories (kcal) per day.
Protein = 525 kcal (1500 x .35)
Carbohydrates = 375 (1500 x .25)
Fat = 600 kcal (1500 x .40)

She would then target the following amount of grams for each macronutrient. Each gram of protein and carbohydrates contains 4 kcal and each gram of fat contains 9 kcal.
Protein = (525/4) = 131 grams (Rounded down from 131.4)
Carbohydrate = (375/4) = 94 grams (Rounded up from 93.75)
Fat = (600/9) = 67 grams (Rounded up from 66.6)

This client would find her better success would be to break these ranges up over 5-6 meals or feedings throughout the day due to low carbohydrate intake.

She would also need to do her best to stay within 5 – 10% of these macronutrient ranges to achieve the best rate of fat loss. Consistency plays a major role in fat loss!

Individualizing Success

Whether you think you are an ectomorph, mesomorph or endomorph, you need to look at the big picture. Do not get overwhelmed attempting to configure the correct macronutrient ranges for your body type. I always recommend that a client look first at their ideal goal set.

Is your main goal fat loss? Then begin with the endomorphic recommendations, weight loss caloric ranges and adjust your meal planning accordingly.

If your main goal is muscle gain, then you may look to start with more of an ectomorphic macronutrient recommendation, weight maintenance or weight gain ranges and adjust as your activity level increases.

For the endurance athlete, you too may want to start with more of an ectomorphic recommendation and adjust according to your training schedule.

We all are different and we all have different training goals. I know that with these strategies in place you will begin to help shape and transform your body in the direction of your personal goal.

About Tyler

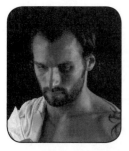

Tyler English prides himself on being a no-nonsense Fitness Professional who is serious about one thing: achieving your results faster than anyone else. Tyler has quickly become Connecticut's leading Fitness Expert. He is the founder of Connecticut's Most Elite Fitness Program, Connecticut Fitness Boot Camp. He is owner of two of Connecticut's Top Personal Training Facilities, Tyler English Fitness in Canton and Tyler English's Fitness Revolution in West Hartford.

Tyler's vision has always been to create a facility that would allow only those seriously committed to creating the lifestyle change that is your personal health and fitness.

That vision has continued to expand as Tyler joined forces with Dr. Joe Klemczewski and became the first Diet Doc Permanent Weight-Loss Program and Clinic in Connecticut. Tyler's fitness industry endeavors didn't stop there, as at the same time, he was selected to become the first Athletic Revolution franchisee in the state of Connecticut. Providing youth fitness and sports performance programming is a natural extension of his commitment to the community.

Tyler is an International Best-Selling Author - he is co-author of *Total Body Breakthroughs* - and his programs have grown to be featured in Shape, USA Today, on Natural Bodybuilding Radio, CT.com, NBC (Connecticut), FOX and WTNH TV, while helping hundreds of busy men and women from all over Connecticut get into the best shape of their lives.

Tyler's work ethic and dedication to goals and a results-oriented lifestyle is apparent in his own body of work. He earned the honor of a Professional Natural Bodybuilder with the World Natural Bodybuilding Federation (WNBF) in only 3 years of competition and won the 2010 WNBF Mid America Lightweight Championship and finished as the 3rd place Middleweight in the World at the 2010 WNBF World Championships. Tyler prides himself on training more like a world-class athlete than your typical gym-going bodybuilder.

In his 8 years in Connecticut, he has helped well over 500 people change they way they look, feel and move. Having worked in the fitness industry for close to a decade, Tyler continuously saw the same thing occurring at gyms and health clubs: people would repeatedly sign a one or two-year membership with the belief that this was the place they were going to get in shape – when the truth was that many of these soon-to-be frustrated exercisers would end up right back where they started.

Tyler has created the "anti health club" environment within each of his facilities and continues to help transform the lives of his clientele.

Tyler has become one of the most respected fitness professionals in the fitness industry – while always displaying a high degree of integrity, responsibility, and ambition. He has proven to be a respected leader within the fitness community, both locally and nationally.

Learn more from Tyler at: www.TylerEnglishBlog.com

CHAPTER 2

Eat More and Stop Exercising
— A 21st Century Approach to Health and Fitness

By John O'Connell

Eat more and stop exercising, sounds appealing and yet slightly confusing, doesn't it?

Why would Ireland's top health and fitness coach recommend such an absurd idea?

The whole concept of eat more and stop exercising is based on the problem that we simply do not eat enough nutritious food these days and have stopped moving as we were born to do. This leads to a host of problems from weight gain and an inability to lose weight, aches and pains in the joints and muscles, all the way up to cardiovascular diseases and cancers.

For the purpose of this book we're going to stick to basic health and weight loss.

Out with the old...

"I know what I need to do." I've heard this statement many times during consultations and general chats.

"Well, why haven't you done it yet?" The reason is because you only think you know what you need to do or what you should do.

And it's based around the outdated theory of eat less and exercise more.

This is a very flawed concept, put less fuel in and demand more energy from the body!!

Also, what sort of notions and fears crop up when you think of eating less and exercising more?

Diets, hunger, restriction, cravings, sacrifice, deprivation, low energy, mood swings, gyms, hard, sweat, uncomfortable, failure, self-consciousness, self-esteem, no confidence, doubt, boredom, no time, effort.

This list is endless and whether you relate to some or all of these, it means you are exactly where the majority of people who start with me are.

STUCK!

They are stuck because they feel it's too hard to diet and restrict and deprive themselves. They don't get going long enough to get great results because they get bored or have so little time to do it. Or they just fear starting and failing again like before.

But it doesn't have to be like this.

Everybody that comes to me has the same fears; they are no different to you or I. But they decided to embrace my concept and run with it.

They decided to eat more and stop exercising. Instead of the usual approach, diet and more exercise, they focused on nourishing their bodies and only did the most effective and efficient forms of training.

So before we go into detail about how to eat more and stop exercising, I need to explain where this comes from and why it works so well.

Eat More simply means eating more nutritious food to feed our body the raw ingredients it needs to function as optimally as we want it to. We need calories to stay alive, we need fat to think, we need carbs for energy, we need protein for repair, we need water to move and we need vitamins and minerals to produce hormones. This is obviously a simplified version of the miracle of life, but it shows that, if we cut out any of the above, things aren't going to run as well as we want them to.

Stop Exercising and start moving and training. Our idea of exercise is walking, running, maybe going to the gym and one of my pet hates 'keeping fit.' This doesn't tie in with what our bodies are actually meant to do.

I have an 18-month-old nephew, Jack. I love watching him play because I'm fascinated by how he moves. He can literally sit on the floor and plant his face between his legs!!

We were born to move, but as we grow up we lose this ability and flexibility unless we actively keep using it. Look at gymnasts, they retain a huge amount of mobility and flexibility simply because they never stop using it.

Moving is much more than walking. Walking actually doesn't require much movement compared to a squat or a gymnastic flip. If it doesn't require as much movement then it doesn't require as much energy. Therefore walking burns very few calories. Don't worry I'm not going to ask you to start jumping and flipping about gymnastics-style, but I am going to show you how to move more so you can ensure you burn more and lose more.

In with the new...

I like to solve things, I always have. I enjoy puzzles, and so whenever I see a problem, I try to solve it or find a better way.

That's the approach I have taken in my career. I see people struggling with weight and health issues and I try to find a better, faster way to solve their problems.

People do question my principles and methods. The fact that I offer a money-back guarantee on all training services doesn't stop that. But if I knew of a way where you could eat junk all day and be in top shape, boy would I use it!!

There are many problems as to why people struggle with weight loss and health.

These are, from what I have identified, the biggest problems we face...

Problem #1: Diets

There is a huge diet mentality that has engulfed us since the 80s and even before. To lose weight we must diet and with that comes deprivation, hunger, mood swings etc.

We start on Monday, fall off the wagon, get back on track, break the diet, start again and so on. This mentality doesn't work. The best way to prove that is to ask anyone who has this mentality: "Are you happy with your current health and body shape?" You'll get a resounding no.

Ask someone who is happy with their current health and fitness levels and they will tell you they never use phrases like this. They are a work in progress, they continue living a healthy lifestyle every day and try to improve constantly, Making small changes often so they never have to 'go on a diet' to get in shape for anything. They are already in shape!

How are you supposed to lose weight or tone up when you feel miserable on a diet?

It's hard! Too hard. How do you fix this problem?

Eat more. Eliminate hunger. Take away restriction and deprivation and you'll be able to follow a plan more easily.

(I'll go in to the exact solutions at the end of the chapter.)

Problem #2: Cravings

Sweet things are nice. Sugar is also very addictive. Certain foods make us feel good when we eat them so when we decide we can't have these, then we start to crave them. We want them more because we can't have them. You'll tell yourself no chocolate for a month, I can't have chocolate, don't even think about chocolate. Guess what? You'll want more chocolate. While studying NLP (Neuro-Linguistic Programming), I learned that one of the fundamental laws of psychology is: we will always get more of what we focus on.

If I tell you not to think about a pink, yellow-spotted lion, you have to actually think about one not to think about it. And even though you've never seen a pink, yellow spotted lion before, at least I hope not, you can actually still picture one in your mind. This shows that you will always get more of what you focus on.

So every time you try not to think about chocolate or whatever you are craving, you are actually making your craving bigger and stronger.

How to fix this problem? Feed yourself foods that actually reduce cravings such as good fats.

Allow yourself to have all the foods you want, but only if you meet certain requirements. Swap the I can't have or I'm not allowed this to I can have this when… and you'll free yourself from your cravings for good.

Problem #3: No time

We live in a world where everything seems to have been made easier for us. We can buy pre-chopped vegetables, we can communicate with someone across the globe instantly, and we can book a holiday any place we want with the click of a mouse.

However, this seems to have reduced our time rather than increase it. It's one of the biggest excuses I hear.

I don't have time to exercise.

First of all, I want to replace the word exercise with training. Training is a much better word, as I'll explain later.

How to fix this problem:

There are 2 questions I ask here:
— *How much time do you need?*
— *How much time do you have?*

The first is usually the hour a day response. If we follow that and train in a gym then we probably need at least another 10-15 minutes to get changed, showered, etc. Plus we have to travel there and back. So an hours training can easily become two hours.

That's 8% of your day, and considering you spend another third of that day sleeping, that's a lot of time to dedicate.

Well the good news is I have discovered that you don't need to spend an hour each day training. You can, but you don't need to. You only need whatever you can spare. The key is quality not quantity.

Which brings us to the second question:

How much time do you have?

First of all figure out when is the best time for you to exercise. Then ask how much time can you allocate to exercise at this time.

That's how much time you should spend training, for now.

Problem #4: No Energy

For me this was the greatest change I made, I went from having no energy to having a ton of it and I liked it. So do my clients. The funny thing is people don't realize that they have so little energy until you show them how much they can have.

When you have so little energy, it's too hard to get up earlier to train. Coming home, feeling dog-tired after a days work, it's going to be very difficult to drag yourself to the gym. Even when you do train the sessions are generally poor because you simply don't have the energy to put into it.

When we feel tired we reach for the quick energy sources, sugar and caffeine. These make us more tired in the long run and we end up 'addicted' to them. Relying on them to keep us going throughout the day. Try to give these up and you'll suffer cravings, headaches, really low energy and massive mood swings.

How to fix this problem?

By feeding ourselves first. Add in more good foods that will reduce our cravings and help eliminate those headaches. Eat foods that our body relies on to function optimally and that help our energy levels. The food we were meant to live off. Water is another important addition here.

Problem #5: Boredom

This plays a huge part in peoples motivation for eating and training. Once it gets boring people lose interest and generally quit. Eating the same foods over and over gets to you and you just say, screw it, I'm going for pizza!

Even worse is doing the same exercise routine week-in week-out in the gym. Not only is this boring for you, but your body also gets bored as it only progresses by being challenged. Doing the same thing over and over, from a physiological perspective is insane.

In order to get fittER, strongER, leanER, healthiER, there must be progression.

Take this for an example:
If you can run 3 miles in 30 mins, you are fit enough to run 3 miles in

30 mins. In order to get fitter, this must change.

Most people tend to start adding time to their sessions. So they run for 35, 45, 50 mins. That's great, but soon you are going to run out of time (excuse the pun). Most people simply can't just keep doing more and more exercise, it's not practical.

How to fix this problem?

Increase the amount of work we do in a given time, or do it faster. These progressions are far more effective at delivering results than adding more time. This will ensure you have a goal to work towards in each session, rather than doing random exercises.

THE SOLUTION

I. Eat More and Stop Exercising
– Eat more vegetables
– Eat more good fats
– Eat more quality protein
– Drink more water
– Eat more herbs and spices

Focus on these first instead of what not to eat. Sure, cutting out certain foods will be helpful but not if they aren't replaced. That's why I always recommend eating more first. Get your energy up, improve your mood, feel good then you can easily reduce the 'bad' foods and get great results.

To save space in this book, I haven't added the actual plan I use, however it is one of the bonuses that comes with the book and you can access it using this link: http://superfastfitnesscamps.com/group/7dayeatmorediet

II. Stop Exercising and Start Training

Make the shift from 'doing exercise' to following a training plan that has goals and targets for each session. Monitor your progress and ensure you are constantly challenging yourself. Get back to moving more by using all the muscles and joints in your body as they were meant to be used.

Sample Training programme. (Video-accessible using the link above)

Warm up using MMAS – Mobility and Muscle Activation Sequence
Then do:

6 burpees
6 push ups
6 reverse prisoner lunges each leg
6 renegade rows each arm

Continue for 5 minutes of total work. Count how many circuits you get in the 5 mins. So you may get 3 full circuits and complete 2 exercises. 3+2

Rest 2-3 minutes and then repeat, aiming to beat your score: get 1 extra rep and you have improved.

You can change the exercises for different sessions too. Usually, I have 2 different circuits in one session and we do both and then repeat and beat the scores.

Training like this eliminates boredom, it is very time efficient and you constantly progress and ensure you get great results. Couple that with eating more of the foods we were meant to eat, and you will start seeing and feeling some amazing changes.

Eat More and Stop Exercising is a shift in conventional thinking. It's an attitude to take towards your health and fitness. Rather than struggling for energy and dragging yourself through each day, start living. Embrace the fact that we can feed the body to feel far better and get back in shape a lot easier.

Nourish Your Body and Start Training!

About John

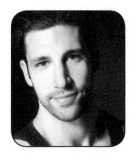

John O'Connell is an International Best Selling Author and one of Ireland's leading health and fitness experts. Having extensive experience working as a personal trainer in a wide variety of gyms in Ireland and abroad, John has trained thousands of clients and has also developed many advanced training programmes for fitness staff.

John is regularly featured on Irish Television as a resident health & fitness expert. He is also sought after for radio, newspaper and magazine features. John has worked as a health and fitness consultant for Lyons Tea and SPAR, the world's largest retail chain. In 2010, he co-authored the International Bestselling book, Total Body Breakthroughs with some of the world's leading health and fitness professionals.

He has an impressive client list, which boasts a number of celebrities and professional organizations including the Irish Police Force and the New Zealand All Blacks.

As well as working with the NZRFU, he has also been involved with many other professional sporting teams, including the Ireland A Senior Rugby Team, the European Cup-winning Leinster Senior Rugby Team, the Dublin Football Team, Queensland Reds Rugby Team, Murphy and Gunn/Newlyn (a Continental Irish Cycling Team) and the Australian Cycling Team, FRF Couriers.

Along with his numerous exercise and health qualifications, John is a licensed Neuro-Linguistic Programming (NLP) Master Practitioner and Life Coach. He is a level 2 internationally certified Strength and Conditioning Coach through PICP, and is one of Ireland's few Bio Signature Modulation practitioners.

John walks his talk. He remains in peak physical condition throughout the year and is a former cyclist. He also auditioned with 10,000 others for a contender's role on the UK TV series Gladiators. He was chosen in the top 16 to compete on the show and only a neck injury prevented him from taking it further.

John's ability to motivate and inspire others is outstanding. He has helped transform the lives of others not just through training but also through his unique style of mental training using his NLP coaching skills.

By combining physical, mental and nutritional training, John can offer a truly unique service to his clients, one that is matched by none. He constantly strives to learn more by attending seminars and internships with world experts so he can help more people achieve the fitness, health and body that they desire.

To avail of John's services, please use the websites below:
www.sffitnesscamps.com – Outdoor Fitness Camps
www.newenergy.ie – Personal Training
www.dublinbootcamps.com - Blog
To contact him, email: john@newenergy.ie

CHAPTER 3

Why Women Store Fat In The Lower Body And What To Do

By Paul Mort

I've personally worked with a LOT of women in my time as a fat loss expert and this has to be the Number 1 ITEM that I've come across the most – accumulation of fat around the gluteals and thighs. In other words – 'fat ass' syndrome! It's important to say here that this is only relative if you're fairly lean everywhere else and you have problems with fat and cellulite in the buttock and thigh areas.

A J-Lo butt might be the 'must have' beach accessory this summer, but all the ladies I work with find it a great source of frustration. I've literally met females with 6-pack abs yet who still carry a fair bit of stubborn fat around the rear!

Why does this happen?

Well the source of this 'stubborn' fat is the female hormone estrogen. We all make estrogen, even men can create it (think man boobs or 'moobs') but it's what happens to it once it's been produced that matters. More importantly, the amount of man-made estrogens (named xenoestrogens) has increased frighteningly in the past 30 or so years.

Did you know for instance that the following things can actually mimic estrogen INSIDE your body from the OUTSIDE? The list includes plastic Bottles, Birth Control Pills, Teflon Coating and commercial meat injected with hormones (most of the meat in your supermarket!).

Now not only are those xenoestroegens (man-made estrogen) a huge problem, it's the body's, or the livers job, to detoxify both of these and excrete them in one-way or another.

Whilst the liver tries to detoxify estrogen to eliminate it from the body it sends it via the bloodstream to the local adipose tissue (fat stores) - in the case of females, this is in the lower body.

Toxins Waffle

Let me break this down a little further for you, when we consume foods that are toxic in nature or difficult to digest, the liver has to work hard in order to break those toxins down and then help to excrete them from the body.

When we're overloaded with these toxins, the liver cant keep up, so the body, being the amazing thing that it is, OBVIOUSLY doesn't want those toxins in the blood stream. Hence, it sends them to the adipose tissue (fat stores) to be stored as fat.

What's that got to do with 'less ass,' Paul? Why is this only in women? How come men get off 'Scot-Free?'

It comes down to liver again, I'm afraid. The liver (an AMAZING organ by the way) produces things called Sex Hormone Binding Globulins (SHBG for short- there's NO WAY I'm typing that out every time I say it). One of the jobs of these SHBG's is to go out and deal with excess estrogen and 'clean it up' – i.e., get rid of it.

NOW.... (You're still with me... right?) Because the liver is so busy dealing with all the other stuff (bad food, bad air, stuff we put on our skin, etc., etc.) it can't deal with producing SHBG'S too!

Now obviously, we don't want that excess estrogen just floating around our bodies, right? So again, it's sent to the fat stores. BUT, in females, there seems to be a LOT of evidence showing that the fat cells in the LOWER body are extremely receptive to storing estogen. Therefore - this should all make sense!

Now that I've got all of the boring stuff out of the way (I'm actually fascinated by it all), lets get onto an action plan.

I should point out that I could write a WHOLE book based on the following, but for the purpose of this just trust me.

1. For 14 days MINIMUM, I need you to removed the following foods from your diet: Wheat (and gluten), Sugar, Dairy, Processed Food, Artificial Sweeteners and Alcohol.

2. Eat a LOT (DO NOT count calories) of fresh fish, organic beef, chicken and turkey, vegetables and fruit.

3. Detoxify estrogen levels by consuming A LOT of vegetables high in Indole-3-carbinol. Watercress is the number one choice here as well as broccoli, cabbage, and cauliflower

4. You can also get indole-3-carbinol in supplement form, although I prefer it in its natural state in food.

5. DO NOT microwave food as it destroys 97% of the flavanoids than can help get rid of this excess fat. Oh, and boiling destroys 66% - that means STEAM!

6. Organic Flax Seed HULLS are great for speeding up the 'excretion' process. Take one teaspoon mixed with water upon waking.

7. Make sure you lift your weights - a resistance training plan of 10-15 reps, 3 sets with short rest periods of 30 seconds is VERY effective. Choose compound movements such as squats, lunges and pushups. If you're doing the three things listed above, you will NOT bulk up.

8. Make sure to drink as much clean, filtered water as you possibly can.

9. You must get off your 'fat ass' to lose your 'fat ass'.

There you have it, my guide to dropping bodyfat safely and effectively from the lower body. You can either read this, nod your head and think "that's nice," OR you can take massive action and get a massive result.

Either way, if nothing changes – nothing changes!

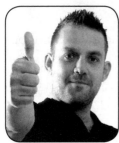

About Paul

Paul Mort is the owner of thefitnesscamp.co.uk and is widely regarded as the UK's leading fat loss expert.

Paul tours the UK teaching other trainers how to get incredible results for their clients who have usually tried everything and failed. He's spoken at the world's biggest fitness convention and has been a nutritional advisor to several premier league footballers.

Paul is the creator of 'the-unstoppable-fat-loss-formula,' a unique fat-destroying system that's proven to work time and time again, regardless of what you've tried before.

You can read more about Paul via:
http://thefitnesscamp.co.uk and
http://paulmort.co.uk

CHAPTER 4

Putting Weight Loss Theory into Practice and Maintaining the Results in a Balanced Way

By Tim Saye – London

The world is full of information about how to lose weight and get in shape fast. Much of it is common sense: everybody who has ever set foot in a gym - and even everybody who chooses to walk on past instead - knows the end result is achieved through a combination of 'eating right' and 'exercising well.' The challenge for most of us, though, comes in applying solid, successful meaning to those words and then taking the steps to act on them accordingly.

The current method used by the majority of the most successful trainers is a combination of resistance and metabolic training coupled with a diet that cuts out processed foods, sugars, starchy carbohydrates, alcohol, and in many cases dairy and even fruit. Without going deeply in to the pros and cons of this method, all I will say for now is that it works to reduce fat for 90% of the population, and works well. I should at this point add that integrating the above with more relaxing pastimes such as Yoga, Massage, Kinesiology and Tai Chi can be very beneficial for balancing hormones, flexibility and clearing the mind. Adding any of these to your routine can only help in the creation of a balanced, healthy and lean body.

The purpose of this chapter is to outline ways that these training and dietary methods can be applied to real life, when other things like work, family, friends, etc. can provide distractions, and then how to easily maintain the results.

Incorporating weight-loss theory into real life.

Let's start with the exercise. Most of the advice out there recommends 3-6 training sessions a week. From personal experience I have found that in general the most efficient results for women come from two sessions of combined resistance and metabolic work and three shorter metabolic sessions per week, while men respond best to three to four resistance sessions and one to two focussing on the metabolic. Incorporating this in to your schedule is best done by simply being consistent: find a time that works well for you and stick to it. Write your training sessions into your diary - once written down the time is put aside and you now have an appointment to train; honour that appointment and you will be rewarded by that feeling of pride that comes with taking a step toward achieving your goals and improving your health.

If time is short do not worry, metabolic sessions should only take 20-35 minutes and can be done anytime, anywhere: shuttle runs in the garden can be very effective, for example. The resistance and combined sessions will usually be a little longer but time can be made: get up an hour earlier, take a lunch-break workout or get to the gym straight after work. Even with a really hectic work week these longer sessions can be squeezed in by simply scheduling them for the weekend; don't worry about lifting weights on consecutive days – whatever your local fitness instructor may tell you, it is not the end of the world.

Once in the routine, exercise should be easy to incorporate into your everyday life. However, breaks such as holidays inevitably crop up and can cause problems. Rest assured most hotels have gyms with some useful equipment in them for resistance sessions and metabolic sessions are easy, using the beach for running, the sea for swimming or, for the winter sports enthusiast, the slopes for skiing. When gyms are not available, skilfully-planned resistance sessions can be done using nothing but your body weight and some props in your room. Writing such a routine falls outside the scope of this chapter, but you will be able to find one on my website at: www.timsaye.com.

Now the harder bit – food. For the purpose of this chapter I will use as an example the current trend of eating meat, fish, eggs, vegetables, some fruit as well as a few seeds and nuts. The principles, though, can be applied to any fat loss eating method. One key to success here is organisation. Breakfast is easy as the day starts at home. You may need to get up a touch earlier to prepare it but scrambled egg, spinach and nuts in a non-stick pan takes 5 minutes and will provide a great start to the day. Daytime snacks and lunch can be a little tougher if you are out and about. A great way to go is to prepare them before you leave for the day. Some people choose to do this in the morning. The snacks can be quite simple – grab a few carrots, some nuts and maybe an apple and off you go. Lunch will sometimes need further preparation but some meat on the grill while you eat your breakfast and a quick salad shouldn't take too much work once you get into the rhythm of things.

If though, like many people, mornings are a bit of a rush and you don't want to sacrifice valuable sleep time preparing your lunch, then other options are available. Many of my clients simply prepare extra for supper the evening before and pop it in a container to take for lunch. Another idea is what Dr John Beradi refers to as the Sunday ritual: putting aside a couple of hours on Sunday to buy food, then cook your meat and chop all the veggies ready for much of the week ahead so it is all there and ready to go when you are. Sometimes you may not be able to do these things, or just forget your food for the day, but all is not lost - a quick trip to the nearest decent supermarket and all kinds of readily available options are there that fit well into the plan - cooked prawns, bagged salads, spinach, ham, sliced turkey or chicken breasts, cooked chicken pieces, nuts, seeds, any kind of fruit or vegetable; these are all available and ready to eat.

Other problems are often presented by eating out. Restaurants can throw temptations into your path, but by asking for a few more vegetables instead of the pasta, rice or potatoes and not overdoing the creamy sauces, you will go a long way to sidestepping them. And the staff should be happy to oblige; after all, part of any restaurant's mission is customer service.

So these are the guidelines that will help you slim down. But losing weight is one thing, keeping it off is another problem entirely: a recent study suggested that a staggering 96% of the population cannot maintain the results in the medium and long term. Maintenance is far less glamorous so often gets neglected. In truth, it is really quite easy, but not many people know how to do it. I will share with you a method I may use with a client after a 6-week fat-loss blast. I'm a huge believer in individualisation, so there will be a few choices for you to make, but the guidelines remain consistent.

Maintenance of your results

Having achieved the lean, toned body that you want, it's time to find the compromise of bringing in a few more of those things you enjoy whilst keeping that new beach-ready body all year round. To start with, it is worth looking briefly at the mind and what is known as the triad of health. The triad of health illustrates the connection between the emotional, the physical and the biochemical. For example - the physical (in this case how you look) affects the emotional (how you feel about your new look), which in turn affects the biochemical (lowered stress hormones, etc.) Simply put, any effect on one is carried through to the others. Sometimes the biochemical can be the priority – sluggish thyroid or slow fat or sugar metabolism – which in turn can affect the emotional and physical. For this reason, I get my clients biochemical balance tested and optimised as a part of any fat-loss package.

Back to the emotional – slip ups happen! People will occasionally miss a training session, eat a pizza or have one too many glasses of wine. This can be followed by the 'Well I've messed up now so I may as well just carry on, have more wine and add in some cake' – the emotional leading to a physical action. This is then often followed by a further sugar craving the next day (the biochemical) and the feeling of 'I've done it once so what the heck' (the emotional). All resulting in guilt and a feeling of hopelessness that can lead again to food and eventually ending up back at square one.

This is where two very important things come in: a positive attitude, and the art of forgiving yourself for indiscretions. Simply do your best to eat well and complete your training sessions, and if you do slip up forgive yourself and get back on track at the next opportunity.

Now we return to the practical skill of maintenance. Once again I'm assuming the fat was lost using a tough diet of vegetables, meat, fish, eggs, nuts, seeds and maybe some fruits, while training was done roughly 5 times per week for optimal results. This is where you need to start making some decisions. Think to yourself what is easiest about this lifestyle? What do you find really hard to do? What things do you miss most from the life you led before? For you to keep this new body and live a great life these questions will have to be answered and addressed.

If you find the training boring, then this can now be adapted. While it has been shown to be a poor way to lose fat in short time periods, aerobic training has been empirically proven to keep fat off a slim body very effectively. This means activities like dance or a favourite class become effective tools in your maintenance arsenal. Most people could then cut down to just two half hour resistance training sessions per week to maintain muscle mass, which is vital for a fast metabolism and lean body. If it's the number of hours you train that bothers you, but the type of training is fine, then most people can come down to 2-3 effective training sessions per week, which should be done gradually over a period of a few weeks.

Many people won't have a problem with the training and will even enjoy it, but do find the food restrictions hard. These people can gradually re-introduce the foods that have been lost from their lives in roughly the following order:
1) Berries
2) Other fruits,
3) Full fat natural yogurts with live culture
4) Red Wine
5) Cheese
6) Starches (sweet potatoes, beans, oats)
7) Other grains and
8) Occasional favorite treats

Foods should be re-introduced one at a time. While I always recommend clients be checked for allergies and intolerances in my practice in order to save time, effort and guesswork, the gradual re-introduction of food types can be a great way to indicate intolerances in your body; as you bring them back they may cause nausea, bloating, headaches, wind or a reaction of any kind like a rash. These foods should be eliminated once again.

Many people will, if the food is re-introduced gradually, be able to maintain a lean body with training 2-3 times a week and including all of the foods listed above. The key guidelines to get to this point would be to introduce one food group one week, then to drop a training session the next, and another food the one after that until you find the point that best suits you. Just be aware that the more and the harder you train, the more foods you can include, even the treats, and vice versa - the less you train, the less foods and treats you can include.

A very important point in maintenance is to keep measuring yourself, keep getting on the scales, pick a favourite dress or shirt and trousers that fit you at your ideal shape and try it on regularly. If you have access to it, get your body-fat percentage checked regularly so you can find out quickly if the fat starts to return and then move back one stage to your true maintenance level. If the fat is not coming back then keep going until you feel you have the perfect balance of life, health and leanness.

As you will hopefully have seen, the key to long term success is not only about getting the right information, but also incorporating it comfortably into your lifestyle. Once you manage that, it becomes easy to achieve and permanently maintain a lean body, great health and true Equilibrium.

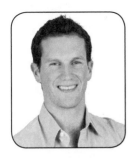

About Tim

Tim Saye – London

Tim has been educated across four continents by the world's leading fat loss, nutrition and strength & conditioning coaches. He pieces this knowledge together into personalised systems that get incredible results.

Tim is an specialist in creating lean, healthy bodies: his expertise lowers injury potential, improves wellbeing and changes bodies for life in remarkably short periods of time. What separates Tim from the handful of other world class personal trainers in the UK is the consistency of his results and the ease with which they are achieved. Everyone who works with him gets from where they are to where they want to be quickly, and they maintain the results easily.

To learn more about Tim and see his tips on fat loss training and nutrition then please visit: www.timsaye.com.

CHAPTER 5

Are your Hormones Making You Fat?

By Graham Webb & Steve Butters

You have probably never been asked this question before, and have probably never asked yourself this question. However, it may be the most important question you ask yourself if you want to lose weight, blast stubborn fat, increase energy and feel great.

Have you tried every diet going without results? Are you sick of pounding away on the treadmill with nothing to show for it? Do you feel like that stubborn fat just will not budge? Are you sick of feeling tired? Are you feeling stressed? Will those cravings just not go away? Are you close to giving up?

Now if you answered yes to any of these then you are not alone. In fact, most people are in the same boat and the problem is getting worse. Why?

Out-of-balance hormones can play havoc with your weight! Your hormones may be the 'silent saboteurs' causing diets and exercise to fail and making you feel like you're the only one who can't lose weight... but the truth is, the causes of your weight-gain can be REVERSED and your hormones can easily be balanced.

Let me tell you about our clients Dave and Rosemary – who you may relate to straight away:

Dave and Rosemary came to us desperate for help. They had tried all the diet and exercise programs they could get their hands on. They had read all the magazine articles telling them the 'secret' weight loss and fat-busting formulas – only to read a completely opposite 'secret' 2 weeks later. They found themselves losing a little bit of weight then putting it all back on - plus a bit extra on top! They both felt tired, nothing was working and the body fat just seemed to creep up and up.

– Dave's health became a major concern – he had 'crept up' to a scary 31+stone, with a huge portion of that fat finding itself stuck on his mid section. If things didn't change soon, his health was going to suffer greatly.

– Rosemary's body fat was getting her down and she was feeling depressed - it seemed to be all accumulating around her thighs, buttocks and navel areas, and no matter what she did… it just wouldn't budge.

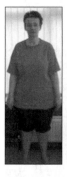 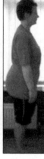 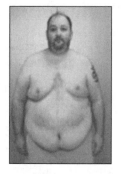

As you can see, a lot of body fat is being stored around her hips, buttocks and thighs.

Dave, at 31 stone, with a lot of his body fat being stored around his midsection.

All, or parts of this story are commonplace in the world today, and that's because we are exposed to so many different types of stressors on the body that all contribute to hormonal imbalance, leading to fat storage.

Let's look at the stress response of the body for today's typical person like Dave or Rosemary:

When we talk about stress, most people think of the typical mental stress of deadlines, work, traffic jams, arguing, feeling out of control, worrying, etc… but this is only 1 of 5 major stressors on the body. The others are:

Physical stress – over/under-exercising, aches & pains, poor posture, injury, poor sleep.

Chemical stress – synthetic chemicals, pesticides, fertilizers, general pollution.

Electromagnetic stress – over-exposure to sunlight, microwave ovens, computers (late at night), telephones, TV, mobile phones, radiation.

Nutritional stress – over/under-eating, consuming processed/artificial foods, yo-yo dieting, poor food choices, sugar, refined carbohydrates, etc...

All of these stressors create an all-too-familiar picture for men and women:

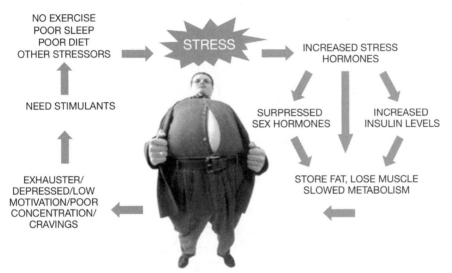

Stress comes in any of the forms mentioned above (nutrition and mental stress being very big stressors throughout most people's days). This leads to an increase in the stress hormone: cortisol.

Cortisol

Cortisol is the hormone of energy and we need cortisol (in bursts) to survive – think 'fight or flight'. However, in today's society, cortisol production is too high and too frequent. When *Cortisol* stays in your blood longer than necessary, as in most people's modern lives, it can have a negative impact on your health.

When your body is constantly producing an abnormally high amount of Cortisol, or there is prolonged exposure to it, your normal pattern is disrupted. Since this hormone is responsible for providing you with energy, it also stimulates the metabolism of carbohydrates and fats – which can increase blood sugar. With this increased level of blood sugar, the excess becomes stored as fat. This is because Cortisol also helps your body re-

53

lease another hormone – **Insulin** (which we will talk about next). These internal activities can lead to an appetite increase. So the longer cortisol is at work in your body, the more hunger pangs you are likely to feel.

Another main issue with Cortisol is that it encourages *fat deposits to accumulate around your stomach*. Therefore, *cortisol trains your body to store fat* more effectively, particularly in your abdominal area.

Insulin

Along with the cortisol response just mentioned, the powerful hormone Insulin is released when you eat sugary foods (cakes, biscuits, sweets, ice cream, etc...) and many starchy carbohydrates (such as white bread, white pasta, white rice, potatoes, cereals etc..). This is because the body's blood sugar levels are raised. It's dangerous for the body to have high blood sugar levels, so it sends insulin along to reduce the blood sugar – very clever! However, insulin takes this blood sugar and stores a lot of it somewhere where we have an unlimited amount of storage space – *THE FAT CELLS. Yes, insulin is a fat storage hormone.*

As if that wasn't bad enough, it also tells the body not to burn any fat because there are still some sugar molecules running round the body ready to burn for energy. Bottom line – *INSULIN TURNS ON FAT STORAGE and TURNS OFF FAT BURNINIG.*

Oh, and one last thing that insulin (along with cortisol) does, is to makes us crave even more of the sugary foods that got us into the fat-storage mess in the first place!

The combination of cortisol and insulin, increased amounts of stress, poor food choices and overall lifestyle throws up another fat-storage issue, and that is one relating to Oestrogen hormones.

Oestrogen

An imbalance of these hormones will also cause *fat storage* (amongst other health problems)! In women, an oestrogen imbalance causes the fat storage to accumulate around the thigh and buttocks areas, and no matter what you seem to do, this 'problem area' does not want to go away. In men, the increased oestrogen that is so common today, results in fat storage in traditional female areas such as the chest, thighs and buttocks, and there is even a term for this increasing phenomena – MOOBS (or man boobs)! Increased oestrogen also lowers the amount of testosterone which is the exact opposite of what men need for strength, muscle building, energy and sex drive!

This oestrogen dominance is a problem! It can cause weight gain, cellulite, some female cancers, a slower thyroid, slower metabolism, bloating, anxiety, brain fog, low sex drive, and poor blood sugar control... Unfortunately, we are living in an increasingly estrogenic society; processed foods, soy products, alcohol consumption, birth control pills, plastics (think food packaging and water bottles), dairy and sugary foods all contribute to the increase in the bad estrogens that can cause weight gain.

This whole hormonal mess causes a cycle of events that self-perpetuates and follows the pattern in the diagram above. The stress, insulin, oestrogen and testosterone imbalance causes weight gain, muscle loss and a *slower metabolism!* This, in turn, leads to feelings of tiredness, mood swings, cravings, energy lows, low motivation leading to poor food choices, and becoming reliant on stimulants for energy, lack of adequate sleep; all leading to an increased stress response – and then the cycle starts again. It's for these reasons that so any people cannot seem to shift the weight regardless of what they try.

What really needs to shift is the hormonal balance. When this happens amazing results will follow – just look at Rosemary and Dave:

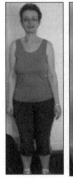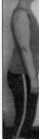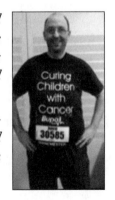

Rosemary lost well over 5 stone and is still going strong. You can see the shape of her hips, buttocks and thighs have really changed as we detoxified and balanced her oestrogens.

Dave has lost over 13 stone and totally changed his shape. The cortisol and insulin producing mid-section has disappeared. (1 stone = 14 lbs)

WOW! Amazing results, I'm sure you will agree!

Both Rosemary and Dave had huge hormonal imbalances that needed looking at, in detail, to truly get the amazing results they dreamed of.

Here's what we did:

- In-depth lifestyle questionnaires, physical assessments and hormonal analysis using the BioSignature Method (from Charles Poliquin) were carried out. From this, an individual nutrition program was developed using foods that built health, burned fat and helped to balance hormones.

- We created a supplementation program that gave the body what was needed to quickly balance hormones and get the body working efficiently again.

- We created a specific FAT BUSTING exercise program tailored to each one of them to give maximum benefits in the shortest time.

Very quickly, amazing results began to show:
Their energy levels soared to levels they had never felt before.
They experienced a full night's sleep for the first time in years.
Their moods and depression lifted and as we began to balance out the tangled web of hormones.
They started stripping weight - FAST!

So, how can you get amazing results like Dave and Rosemary? How can you blast fat off your thighs, buttocks and belly? How can you get the body and health you deserve?

It's actually a lot simpler than you might think.

Here are the top 10 ways you can control your hormones instead of letting them control you (and your fat)!

1. Cut out all sugar and simple carbs to keep insulin levels down. Avoiding insulin spikes is simply the key to preventing 'storage mode.'

2. Increase your protein intake. Protein is needed for keeping insulin levels down, turning on the fat-burning hormones, building lean tissue, making you feel fuller for longer and providing important vitamins and minerals found mostly in animal produce. Great sources include all oily fish, chicken, turkey, wild or naturally- reared meat and free range eggs.

3. Increase your vegetables. Green vegetables really are super foods. They are packed full of vitamins and minerals essential for optimal hormonal balance. They are the best source of low GI carbohydrates

(along with fruits), great sources of fibre and their oestrogen-reducing properties cannot be over-emphasized. Increase your greens to decrease those thighs.

4. **Eliminate processed foods.** Quite simply, processed foods are not good for your health, your weight or your hormonal response. If you can't understand or spell any of the ingredients on the list, then put it back on the shelf. Another way of thinking about it would be to ask yourself if it was around 10,000 years ago. If it was, then the chances are it will be good, if it wasn't then it's probably best to leave it where you found it. Stick to whole natural foods that promote health.

5. **Exercise 4 - 5 times per week.** This seems like a no brainer and it is, but the type of exercise is important. Whilst any exercise is better than sitting on your backside, there are ways to really ramp up the fat loss. The most important part of your exercise program should be based around resistance training (i.e. using weights – yes, especially women!). You need to build lean tissue to burn fat and balance hormones. For every 1 pound of lean tissue you build (which is about the size of a small strawberry), you will burn an extra 50 calories per day!

6. **Eat regularly throughout the day.** Eating smaller meals more frequently will keep blood sugar stable, and therefore avoids the insulin spikes that cause fat storage and carb cravings.

7. **Drink lots of water** and avoid any other calorie-laden drinks. Increasing your water alone will have significant impacts on energy and fat loss. Sugary drinks and even sugar-free drinks should be banned, as they will perpetuate the insulin-fat storage cycle. Caffeine should also be limited as this can increase cortisol. 1 to 2 cups per day should be the maximum and definitely not after 3:00 p.m.

8. **Get a good night's sleep!** Many people do not get enough high quality sleep and this can be a major factor as to why they cannot lose weight. Many hormonal processes take place during the deeper stages of sleep,which aid weight loss, so this is an essential part of the jigsaw puzzle to get right. Avoid caffeine in the late afternoon and evening. Avoid watching TV in bed or doing any computer work late at night as this stimulates the stress hormone cortisol, which affects sleep quality, and will then affect many other physical and mental regeneration processes, thereby hampering your success.

9. **Reduce stress.** Relaxation is key for weight loss! As you now know, stress can cause high levels of Cortisol to be present and when this happens more abdominal fat is stored. Introduce relaxation classes, or tai chi to help with the stresses of daily life. Do more things with family and friends – play with the kids, book days out, listen to your favourite piece of music, go to the cinema. All too often we get caught up in daily life and forget what makes us happy and relaxed. The key is to plan these things, put them into your schedule and make time for yourself.

10. **Supplement your diet.** Adding high quality supplements to your diet will fast-track your results and accelerate the fat loss process. Everyone would benefit from adding certain supplements to their diet to help untangle the hormonal web. At the very least, a good multivitamin and omega 3 should be added to your diet. To get specific about which supplements will help you and your hormones the most, you would need a full assessment with a trained practitioner, but this is great place to start.

If you follow these 10 rules we guarantee that you will lose fat and regain hormonal balance.

Here is a quick start guide to help you decide which hormonal category is dominant in your life:

HORMONE	FAT STORAGE	IMPLICATIONS	SOLUTIONS
Cortisol	Belly and midsection	Feeling wired but tired. Wake up tired. Sleep problems. Feeling stressed. Always on the go. Irregular bowel activity.	Introduce meditation, tai chi, or relaxation sessions to your week. Reduce alcohol. Eat regularly.
Insulin	Love handles and upper back	Mid-morning and mid-afternoon energy slumps. Sugar/carb cravings.	Reduce starchy carbs. Eat every 3-4 hours with protein included in the meal/snack. Increase consumption of fats.
Estrogen	Hips, thighs and buttocks	Mood swings. Lethargy. Bloating and wind.	You need to detoxify. Green vegetables need to be increased. Avoid soy, dairy and sugary foods and increase fibre intake

A more in-depth analysis is needed but this should give you an idea. To receive a more in-depth analysis, contact info@easyfitpt.co.uk

It is not common practice to get our hormones checked, but even the slightest imbalances can tip the scales and just make weight-loss a futile exercise, which is why it is a great idea to see someone like the Easyfit personal training team to find out just how you can tailor your program to give you the body of your dreams.

Hormones are often not integrated into diet programs because, frankly, they are very complex. There are numerous different hormones in the body, and these present over a thousand possible combinations that can affect your health and weight.

So, to answer the question 'Are your hormones making you fat?'

YES! But now you know how to change that and make them work for you.

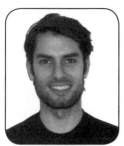

Steve Butters

About Steve and Graham

Steve Butters and Graham Webb are the founders of the UK's fastest growing personal training company, Easyfit Personal Training.

Having spent 10 years at the forefront of health and fitness in the UK, Steve and Graham now lead a team of some of the top trainers in the country.

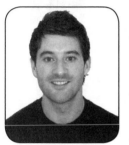

Graham Webb

Starting from Sport & Exercise Science degree backgrounds, they have studied under the world's leading experts on health, nutrition, strength, fitness and lifestyle coaching. The number of qualifications gained over this time period is extensive, giving them all the tools they need to get the best results.

They have been featured in both the local and national press, along with regularly writing for health and wellness magazines such as *Zest, Closer, Body Confidential, Live Cheshire* and *THE magazine*. They have also appeared on local and national TV and are trusted by some of the country's top celebs and sports stars to get them into shape.

Easyfit operates mainly throughout the North of the UK, and if anyone wants guaranteed results like Dave and Rosemary, then you can contact us at: info@easyfitpt.co.uk

Website – www.easyfitpt.co.uk

CHAPTER 6

The Simplest Most Effective Nutrition Plan

By Trevor Buccieri

There are always exceptions to any rule, but in general all people are built the same. So why then do so many struggle in our country with extreme weight problems? Throughout my training career, I have encountered countless questions, but by far the absolute winner above all is, "What should I eat?" Although a completely valid and straightforward question, there truly is no one answer that will work for all people. Everyone in their mind already has a continuing menu of their 20 favorite foods, which seem to rotate and repeat on a shuffle – over and over again. Yes, people do want to learn the perfect menu that will get them in the best shape of their lives, but at the same time, people are afraid of change; especially extreme and restricted changes. Well, rest assured, I have great news for you that begins with our opening statement. All people are built the same. Therefore, the principles that work for one will ultimately work for another. What will separate people are simply the food choices they decide to apply to these principles throughout the day.

Now I have heard countless excuses as to why someone can't possibly eat healthy – ranging from "I don't have time" to "work is too busy," and "I have kids, it's too hard," or "it takes too much time," etc. All true, but what it really comes down to is, do you truly want to make a life-altering change? Do you want to be healthy, leading a higher quality of life with more energy and strength, a much clearer mindset, a leaner body with more vitality and vigor, or do you want to remain unhappy with yourself and your body? The truth is that no one has to live with their choices but you. It is 100% your decision. So ask yourself. Are you happy with your health, your nutrition, your body? Are you happy with yourself, or it is time for a change?

What I want to talk to you about is what I like to call – The Simplest Most Effective Nutrition Plan that I know. Yes, there are nutrition plans full of tricks, loopholes, special items that are the magic ingredient for success, blah-blah-blah, but not here. This is the most basic approach that I have used with so many of my clients, with the most success. Here's why: IT WORKS and IT JUST MAKES SENSE... not to mention, it doesn't take a rocket scientist to get started on it today!

Lets talk about fruits and vegetables first. Plain and simple, no one eats as many as you are supposed to when the fact remains that these foods are true super foods. These foods are an amazing source of vitamins, minerals and fiber. They also possess extremely powerful antioxidants and phytochemicals that are proven to fight several chronic diseases such as stroke, type II diabetes, high blood pressure, cardiovascular disease and several forms of cancer. To make it simple, these foods keep your immune system thriving. When eating your fruits and vegetables, it is best to try to get a large variety of color in your selection. Differing color pigmentation in fruits and vegetables represent different nutrients inside these foods, which will help your body in their own way. Therefore, variety is another key.

Red fruits and vegetables contain what is called *lycopene*. Lycopene in tomatoes, watermelon and pink grapefruit, for example, may help reduce risk of several types of cancers, especially prostate cancer. Lycopene in raspberries, red grapes, strawberries, and other fruits and vegetables act as powerful antioxidants that protect cells from damage.

Orange/yellow fruits and vegetables contain **carotenoids**. Beta-carotene in sweet potatoes, pumpkins and carrots is converted to vitamin A, which helps maintain healthy mucous membranes and healthy eyes. It has been reported that carotenoid-rich foods can help reduce risk of cancer and heart disease. It can improve immune system function.

Green fruits and vegetables contain a natural plant pigment called *chlorophyll*. Some members of the green group, including spinach and other dark leafy greens, green peppers, peas, cucumber and celery, contain *lutein*. Lutein may help reduce risk of cataracts and age-related macular degeneration, which can lead to blindness if untreated.

Blue/purple fruits and vegetables contain what is called **anthocyanins**. Anthocyanins in blueberries, grapes and raisins act as powerful antioxidants that protect cells from damage. They may help reduce risk of cancer, stroke and heart disease. Other studies have shown that eating more blueberries is linked with improved memory function and healthy aging.

White fruits and vegetables are colored by pigments called **anthoxanthins.** They may contain health-promoting chemicals such as allicin, which may help lower cholesterol and blood pressure and may help reduce risk of stomach cancer and heart disease. Some members of the white group, such as bananas and potatoes, are good sources of the mineral potassium, too.

Whole grain carbohydrates are also absolutely necessary as they provide your body with essential antioxidants, phytonutrients, fiber, vitamins, and minerals. Not to mention the fact that foods rich in carbohydrates (especially clean carbohydrates) are your body's best source of energy. These foods provide your brain, heart, and nervous system with a constant supply of energy to keep you moving, breathing, and thinking properly. Whole-grain foods are also associated with lowering your risk for several chronic diseases and conditions including heart disease, cancer, diabetes, and gastrointestinal troubles. The key here though is the term "whole grain." This means that the grain has not been tampered with in any way. It has not been refined or enriched. Refining consists of taking a whole wheat kernel and stripping it of its fiber, wheat germ, and bran which contain all of the major nutrients we benefit from with whole grains. What we are left with is starch, which is pretty much white bread containing no true nutrients whatsoever. Back in 1942, the government passed what is called The Enrichment Act. This act required companies refining their products (stripping them of nutrients), to re-enrich them with vitamins and minerals in order to provide consumers with the proper vitamins and minerals that were taken out. So now when you look at the back of any grain or bread products and you see the word "enriched", you know this should not be one of your sources. This is not a whole food. The problem with these foods is that they are completely overeaten by many, which causes neglect from eating many other foods, such as vegetables and fruits, due to being too full. These foods should not be excluded, but do deserve a smaller area on your plate and on your priority list.

Proteins are your building blocks for repairing bodily tissues including your muscular system, ligaments, tendons, blood, your skeletal system, and many other bodily chemicals and hormones. The human body is about 45% protein. It is an essential macromolecule without which our bodies would be unable to repair, regulate, or protect ourselves. Your body uses more energy to assimilate dietary protein, meaning you burn more calories eating protein as compared to carbohydrates and fats. This keeps hunger at bay, and more importantly, prevents drastic spikes in blood sugar, which can lead to bingeing and also a crash in energy. Proteins are involved in virtually all cell functions. They are used as antibodies, which defend the body from antigens (foreign bodily invaders). Proteins are used for the production of muscle contractions and movement. Structural proteins such as *elastin* and *collagen* help provide support for our connective tissues, tendons and ligaments. As enzymes, proteins are used to help the body perform tasks more efficiently – such as the breakdown of *lactose* in milk by the enzyme *lactase*. There are hormonal proteins, which are considered messengers as they help coordinate certain bodily activities. An example of this is insulin's regulation of glucose metabolism through the control and stabilization of blood sugar concentrations. Without proteins, the most basic functions of life could not be carried out. Even something such as breathing requires muscle contraction and muscle contraction requires proteins. It is absolutely essential.

Fats are an absolute necessity in our daily nutrition as well. Not only is it a natural insulator and protector for bodily organs, but it is also a nutrient which helps to lower our cholesterol levels as well as our instances of Cardiovascular Disease. Many of the fats we will be receiving with this nutrition program occur naturally from our protein sources – some of which is saturated fat. Now, it has been scientifically-proven that foods which have naturally-occurring saturated fats such as steak, chicken, eggs, even bacon (as long as it is grass fed, hormone and antibiotic free and free of nitrate preservatives) will not heighten your circumstances for Cardiovascular Disease. In fact, a recent study where participants ate bacon (nitrate free) every day for 6 weeks, actually showed a decrease in arterial cholesterol deposit levels, which is the primary function of an unsaturated fat. The issues of high cholesterol and blood pressure have more to do with the other food choices people are making, such as hydrogenated trans fats found in baked goods, pre-packaged foods, fried foods, margarine, you name it. There are too many foods possessing hydrogenated oils and there lies the real issue.

Here is my ultimate solution for you. The following is what I call *The Simplest Most Effective Nutrition Plan That I know*. It is based on 3 simple rules. Follow it and you are assured absolute success.

The Simplest Most Effective Nutrition Plan That I Know

No more excuses. This is a 3-step nutrition plan that can fit anyone's schedule. Follow this with consistency and you are guaranteed some solid results.

DO NOT FOLLOW IT FOR 2 DAYS, LINGER AWAY FROM IT FOR 3 DAYS, BACK ON 2, OFF 4, ETC. AND WONDER WHY "IT'S NOT WORKING." BE CONSISTENT AND YOUR RESULTS WILL SHINE!

Step 1.) Eat Five meals per day - Eat roughly every 2.5-3.5 hours, trying to make the meals are as evenly portioned as possible.

Step 2.) Eat your foods in THIS SPECIFIC ORDER - First eat 1-1.5 servings of any fruit (go light on the grapes). Also eat 1-1.5 servings of vegetables. Second eat 1 or more servings of lean protein (chicken breast, turkey breast, ground turkey, lean ground beef 93%, salmon, white fish, etc.) MAKE SURE TO EAT YOUR FILL ON THE FRUITS, VEGGIES AND PROTEINS FIRST.

IF AND ONLY IF you are still hungry, then eat your starchy/granular carbohydrates. IF YOU DON'T NEED THEM, DON'T EAT THEM. You want to eat only 100% whole grain starch here (100% whole wheat pasta, 100% long grain brown rice, ezekial or 100% whole wheat bread, sweet potato etc). ONLY EAT A VERY SMALL PORTION SO THAT YOU ARE SATISFIED NOT STUFFED!!

Once you know how much you are consistently eating here from each food category, then you can begin mixing the order of your foods and start preparing some of your vegetable, protein and fruit combination favorites. For example, one thing I love to do is a vegetable stir-fry mixed with chicken and a nice fruit salad on the side. Another thing I love doing is taking a nice fresh bed of spinach greens, slicing up some grilled chicken and fresh fruits and putting it on top. You can then finish this up with a balsamic vinegar and olive oil homemade dressing. This way, I can keep all of my foods in line with the proper portion sizes, and mix it up a bit. It really helps keep things fresh!

Step 3.) AGAIN – Eat every 2.5-3.5 hours. This is great for portion-control here. If you are too stuffed from the last meal at that time, that means you ate too much from the previous meal. If you are starving, you need to eat a little bit more at the previous meal so you are starting to get hungry around that time. YOU NEVER WANT TO BE STUFFED OR HUNGRY. YOU ALWAYS WANT TO BE "GOOD." When increasing or decreasing your serving sizes to accommodate hunger, make sure to always keep the servings in proportion. [50/50 fruits to vegetables, and a solid serving of protein.]

Some Additional Daily Nutrition Tips

- Drink 3/4 of your body weight in ounces of water - Ex. if you weight 100lbs, drink 75 ounces
- Eat 1 Serving of Fat Per Day from 1 of the following sources
- Avocado, 100% Natural Peanut Butter, Nutiva Coconut Oil, Flaxseed Oil, Fish Oil, Olive Oil,

Follow The Food Choices From This List

The Simplest Most Effective Nutrition Plan - Food List

FRUITS	VEGETABLES	PROTEINS	CARBOHYDRATES
Apple	Asparagus	Boneless skinless	Oatmeal
Banana	Cabbage	chicken or turkey	Hummus
Orange	Cucumber	Venison	Lentils
Clementine	Zucchini	Lean Pork Loin	
Grapefruit	Mushrooms	Cottage Cheese	Baked beans (sauce
Watermelon	Squash	Organic Greek Yogurt	drained)
Cantaloupe	Beets		Raw beans (kidney,
Honeydew	Carrots	Fish	soy black, etc.)
Peach	Eggplant	Shellfish	
Pear	String beans	Eggs	Spelt
Tangerine	Bok choy	(Omega 3 Egglands	Barley
Mango	Cauliflower	Best)	Buckwheat
Papaya	Kale		Quinoa
Berries (black, blue,	Peppers	Ham slices	Millet
rasp)	Tomatoes	Red meat lean 93%	Rye
Pineapple	Broccoli	Lean ground turkey	
Prunes	Celery		Ezekial (sprouted
Kiwi	Lettuce	Tuna	grain) products -
Kale	Spinach	White fish	Breads, English muf-
Leeks	V-8 juice	Salmon	fins, pitas, waffles
Strawberries	Brussels sprouts	Protein powder	
Blueberries	Collard greens		100% Long Grain
Apricots	Homemade Marinara		Brown/Basmati Rice
Cherries	Sprouts		
Kiwi	Bell Peppers		100% whole wheat
	Avocado		bagel (no high fruc-
			tose)
			3 (3.6oz) 100% whole
			wheat Pancakes
			100% whole wheat
			English muffins
			100% whole wheat
			Pita
			100% whole wheat
			Tortilla
			100% whole wheat
			Pasta or noodles
			Potato/sweet potato

There you have it. The simplest most effective nutrition plan I know. Basic, yet endless opportunities. Here's to your health and longevity. Thanks much for reading.

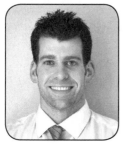

About Trevor

Trevor A. Buccieri, MS, ACSM began his personal training career with his first company, Personal Best Fitness, in May 1998. He has personally trained more than 10,000 personal training sessions. Today, his company has developed into Body & Soul Boot Camp: The Experience, and specializes in corporate wellness, group personal training, and traditional personal training.

Trevor holds a Master's degree in Health and Physical Education (2004) from Canisius College, Buffalo, NY and a bachelor's degree in Exercise Physiology (2002) from State University of New York's College at Brockport, Rochester, NY. Trevor is also an ACSM certified personal trainer (CPT).

He has worked with multiple professional athletes such as Dominique Wilkins of the Atlanta Hawks, Pervis Ellison of the Boston Celtics, Tony Martin of the Atlanta Falcons and Chris Slade of the New England Patriots, as well as non-athletes of all ages and physical abilities.

Trevor has been actively involved in the fitness industry for more than fifteen years as a club manager, owner, personal fitness trainer, and corporate wellness assistant supervisor at Eastman Kodak in Rochester, NY. He has written articles for many publications including The East Aurora Advertiser, The East Aurora Bee Publications, The Buffalo News and The Buffalo News Magazine.

Trevor was an ACE personal trainer instructor for the vocational technology BOCES educational system. His system is tested and proven and combines the three major areas that every business needs to address if they are to see a return on their employee benefits investment: these are exercise, nutrition and action (as in accountability/education).

"Trevor's Body & Soul Boot Camp is the place for you to work out. The program is designed to provide various levels of exercise progressions for each exercise, challenging and pushing everyone to their individual ability levels.

Several of Buccieri's clients have come to the program with serious health problems and each has seen the number of prescription drug medications prescribed to them eliminated or drastically reduced in just months.

After working with Body & Soul, its easy to see, if you're looking for a washboard stomach or to recover mobility in your lower back after an accident – If you work for it, you'll get it. The proof is in the results."

- Timothy Chipp, Editor - East Aurora Bee Publications, *Boot Camp Replaces The Gym*, August 2010

CHAPTER 7

Fitness and Weight Loss for Baby Boomer Women

By Becky Williamson

By definition, we are women born during the post World War II Baby Boom (between 1946 and 1964). So, all of us are now well over 40, and some of the early boomers are entering their mid-sixties. We "boomers" have many different roles: mother, wife, grandmother, working woman, retired woman, caregiver to grandchildren, caregiver to aging parents — we're a diverse group with regard to where we are in our lives. What we do share with each other whether we're raising kids or babysitting grandchildren, working full time or in retirement—is that our bodies are changing. This doesn't have to be a bad thing. In fact, I believe that a well-planned exercise program and supportive nutrition can really re-define what "middle age" means.

Sixty or seventy years ago, a woman in her 50's was OLD. Today, we boomers are changing this perception. We can set the example that women do NOT have to become "frumpy" and fat as we approach or exist in this place called "middle age." We're living a lot longer these days, and I submit to you that we might as well feel great and look great while we're here.

Does a Boomer Body Need a Different Workout?

We probably don't need a completely different program, but we women over 40 or 50 do have a few things to deal with that younger women don't yet deal with: hormonal changes, bone density changes, and changes in muscle mass. These three things can wreak havoc on our weight, our posture and our mood if we don't exercise, sleep well or eat well.

Luckily, some of the things we attribute to "aging" are really due to inactivity, poor food choices, and sometimes even poor exercise choices. *If we maintain a sedentary lifestyle, we most certainly will gain fat and lose muscle as we age.* We might have gotten away with over-eating, poor nutrition and not enough exercise in our younger years, but very few of us will get away with it in middle age. This is one of the key differences between us "boomer" women and women much younger than us.

The good news is, we CAN manage the age-related issues we face such as thinning bones, a slowing metabolism and decreased muscle mass. We can be fit and we can look fabulous.

The Boomer Metabolism

So, what happens as we age? Does our metabolic "furnace" just poop out?

Here's what the research says: Adults who don't do any form of muscle strength training lose between 5-7 pounds of muscle every decade. *Muscle tissue is metabolically active—it burns calories.* Therefore, muscle loss results in a lowered metabolism over time. Studies indicate that the average adult experiences anywhere from a 1 to 3 percent reduction in their metabolic rate per decade. Here's the kicker: Most of the drop in metabolic rate older adults experience is from muscle loss, NOT due to the natural aging process!

There are two main reasons that "boomer" women lose muscle:
We're "dieting" junkies
When was the last time you said these words: "I'm dieting" or "I'm on a diet." I hope to convince you to take these statements out of your vocabulary! When we chronically take in way too few calories, our body may resort to breaking down muscle tissue for energy. Because muscle is heavier than fat, we get fooled into thinking we're successful "losers" because we're experiencing such great weight loss on the scale. What we don't realize is that we're lowering our metabolic rate with this chronic calorie restriction nonsense, and this will eventually cause us to put on MORE weight when we return to "regular" eating – and we always do!

We become less active

I often wonder if this is more of a mindset thing than a physical thing for some of us. We get fooled into thinking that as we get to a certain age, it is inappropriate to do certain activities and that we need to "slow down." Frankly, we need to start realizing the truth lies in the exact opposite. We're getting older—time to ramp up our activity! As we become less active, the pounds pile on and our joints take on more stress due to added weight. We then have a harder time moving around—so we become even more sedentary. It's a vicious circle.

The great news is, both these reasons — chronic dieting and a sedentary lifestyle — can be changed! You have complete control over both of these lifestyle choices. Boomer women can and should increase their metabolic rate in order to fight off middle age weight gain. You can do this with simple changes to your current nutrition and exercise habits.

Three Nutrition Tips to Stay Lean After 40

1. Eat often, eat small

You need to eat — and eat regularly — in order to keep your metabolism stoked, stabilize your blood sugar and keep yourself feeling good. I suggest you eat 3 small meals and 2-3 small snacks each day. Eating small meals and snacks more frequently (every 3 to 3.5 hours) provides your body with a regular supply of fuel it needs. Also, your metabolic rate increases just a little bit each time you have a meal (digestion requires energy—calories!), so you elevate your metabolism just a tiny bit each time you eat. Going for long periods without eating, skipping meals completely, or eating large meals less frequently may lead to increased fat storage – all bad for a boomer body.

2. Have some lean protein with every meal or snack

Protein is really important for a boomer body for a number of reasons. Protein digests more slowly than carbohydrate, so it keeps you feeling full longer. Protein is essential in order to supply the building blocks our body needs to manufacture new muscle tissue. And finally, protein adds a little boost to our metabolism because it takes a few more calories to digest. Examples of lean protein include: fish, chicken breast, turkey breast, sirloin, pork tenderloin, eggs/egg whites, low fat cheese, and beans.

3. Don't go "Fat Free"

Many women over 40 are "fat phobic". I think this stems from low-fat diets that were popular in the 80's. Trying to pull out all the fat in your diet is going to backfire (because it's just not going to work long term). It's not a good thing nutritionally anyway — your body needs some fat. A little bit of "good fat" at every meal will help keep you feeling fuller and decrease your chances of binging later on. Examples of good, heart healthy fats include nuts, seeds, nut butters, avocados and olive oil.

Three Exercise Tips to Stay Lean After 40

1. Incorporate full body, multi-joint exercises into your workouts
"Full body" exercises are exercises that involve more than one joint at a time. Examples include squats, lunges, push-ups and pull-ups. These exercises use LOTS of muscles--thereby burning more calories. One of the best benefits of using multi-joint exercises in your workouts (aside from the significant calorie expenditure they create) is that your workout time will end up being much shorter than when you do a traditional "single body part" routine.

Time saving tip....
Instead of resting between several sets of the same exercise, try "super sets": Perform one set of an exercise, and then immediately do another exercise that works a different area on your body (example push ups, then squats). This gives one area of your body a rest while another area is working. Repeat exercises #1 and #2 in succession with little to no rest between the exercises, and then choose two new exercises and do the same thing. By minimizing rest time, you shorten your overall workout time.

Example:– Superset workout: (please see bonus module for a review and explanation of this workout)
A1: Push ups
A2: Hamstring curls on stability ball

B1: Lat pull down
B2: Split squats

C1: Squat-to-press
C2 Overhead triceps extensions

2. FATIGUE your muscles
When working with weights or resistance tubing, make sure the weight or tube you select provides a challenge. This is one of the biggest strength-training mistakes I see in women over 40. Very often I see them in the gym lifting teeny tiny "Barbie" weights. If you are reha-

bilitating a joint or currently have tendonitis, you most certainly want to be very careful and use very light resistance. However, if you are not rehabilitating a muscle or joint—fatigue those muscles!!!! You're not as fragile as you might think.

You absolutely must fatigue your muscles when you strength train in order to generate new muscle tissue.

Aim for 3 strength workouts per week and make sure to take a day of rest in between strength training days, in order to give your muscles a chance to rest and rebuild.

3. Consider INTERVAL cardio workouts in place of lower intensity cardio workouts

Supercharge your calorie expenditure by doing intervals of hard effort interspersed with intervals of moderate effort. Unlike longer, lower intensity bouts of exercise, high intensity interval training provides an increase in metabolic rate after your exercise is completed, helps your body to better utilize stored fat for fuel all day long, and takes less time than traditional "steady" state cardio.

Aim for 3-5 cardio workouts per week, with most of them being "interval" cardio in nature. Remember, high intensity interval training is done for a shorter period of time than traditional "steady state" exercise, so although you'll be working out very hard, it's for a much shorter period of time.

If you're new to interval training, substitute just one interval cardio workout for a "steady state" cardio workout each week and work up from there. Always remember to warm up very well before any workout, but especially before an interval training workout.

Example – High Intensity Cardio workout:
After a 5-6 minute warm up, do the following while walking, running, swimming or while on any cardio machine at your health club:
Do the exercise HARD for 30 seconds
Do the exercise at a low to moderate pace for 1 minute

Repeat this HARD EFFORT/RECOVERY PACE cycle for 4-10 cycles depending on your current fitness level and your available time frame. If you're new to high intensity exercise, start with just 4 cycles on intervals and work up slowly to a maximum of 10 cycles.

After your last cycle, cool down with a low effort for 5 minutes

Time saving tip....
Split up your workouts: Do a cardio interval program right after awakening in the morning and then do your strength work later in the day or in the evening. There are two great benefits to exercising twice a day: Your time commitment per workout is very small (15-25 minutes per session), and you stoke your metabolic rate TWICE in one day!

Final Thoughts

As I mentioned earlier in this chapter, we know for a fact that a lot of the issues some of us experience with regard to "aging" are actually issues related to decreased activity and poor eating habits. These things are totally within your control!! You have in front of you advice and exercises you can use right now to look better, feel better and have more energy! Is there any reason why you wouldn't take advantage of them?

We "Boomer" women have the power to re-define what aging looks like. We have the power to encourage the younger generations to exercise, eat well and take care of their bodies by being role models for them. Think about that: By taking care of our bodies and eating well (and feeding those in our care well) we may actually influence the younger generations in a positive way. This seems like a win-win situation to me!

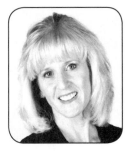

About Becky

Becky Williamson is an exercise physiologist, fitness coach and fitness business owner in Northern California. Armed with a graduate degree in kinesiology, her experience spans over 25 years and includes experience in corporate fitness, personal training and even scientific research (she ran a human physiology lab for the Advanced Life Support Division at NASA-Ames Research Center in Mountain View, CA).

Becky wears many hats in the fitness world. As President of lifeSport Fitness in San Jose, California, Becky and her team provide in-home personal training, fitness boot camps, and corporate fitness programs to Bay Area residents and corporations. Becky also has an online presence at www.beckywilliamson.com where she educates and motivates "Boomer" aged women to make their boomer years their best years through exercise and proper eating.

Becky's philosophy of a "fitness lifestyle" is evident in the programs and products she creates. Her goal is to find creative ways in which to engage her customers in taking an active part in achieving their goals. "It's not just a workout, it's a lifestyle!", she can often be heard saying.

Client testimonials highlight Becky's professionalism, quick wit, and her obvious passion and commitment to her clients' success as reasons for working with her — the fact that she helps them get results might be a reason, too! Whether she's teaching an early morning boot camp, designing a post-rehab program for a customer with a hip replacement, or presenting a motivational lecture at a corporate site, Becky's passion and ability to motivate those around her leaves her clients excited and ready to take action.

In addition to her Master's Degree, Becky is certified as a Health/Fitness Instructor and an Advanced Personal Trainer through the American College of Sports Medicine, and is a Certified Personal Fitness Trainer through the American Council on Exercise. She also holds a certification from the American Academy of Health and Fitness Professionals as a Post-Rehab Specialist.

When she's not working, Becky can often be found cheering at a sporting event for one of her two children or working out at the gym with her husband. She has successfully juggled her roles as businesswoman, wife and mother for many years…and as a lover of adventure travel, has also found time to bungee jump in New Zealand, zip line through the jungle canopy in Belize, swim with the dolphins in Mexico and surf in Hawaii.

CHAPTER 8

How to Develop Hero Focus

By Oliver Chapman

In this Chapter I want to take you to the next level, helping you go beyond where you are now, by showing you how unbreakable focus can help you achieve exactly what you want, and why this is vital for your success.

Because you know, its not all just about having the perfect training program, or the most amazing nutrition plan, its about much more than it, its about what I call hero focus, because that's what I want you to develop. I use a hero as my analogy for this, because if you think of a hero, any hero, they need one thing and its always that one thing which makes them a hero, focus; the focus to never give up and always keep trying. When someone's life is at risk, would you throw in the towel? Of course not, so why do it for anything else in life.

If you had the same focus as a hero for making yourself look, feel and perform at your best, don't you think you would achieve those goals?

You see it's all about your mind-set, and when I say mind-set, what I mean is your focus, getting in the zone and not letting anything stop you. Because to be honest, I'm no different to you reading this book, I can't eat what I want and stay lean, I can't miss workouts often and stay in shape, and for a while I thought that was just how it was.

Until I changed my mind-set, I got focused and realized that all you need to do is know what you want, and most important, believe you can achieve it – better yet, decide you've already done it – sounds too easy, right? … Well, it's really not!

But it is simple, instead of being the person who sits on the side lines, uses an excuse and says that one piece of cake is okay, missing a training session is fine, late nights don't matter and you can recover with no sleep, become the opposite. Decide what you want, and that you will become that person no matter what; you will become your own hero, become the person who never gives up or gives in, the person with unstoppable focus!

That's the focus you need, that unbreakable focus. I'm sure you've seen it in people; all the people who come out on top, the winners that consistently get better, the people who have great businesses, the entrepreneurs have it and when you decide you have it, which can be from right now, nothing can stop you, all you need to do, is think, its the only option! For instance, decide there is no breaking the diet or missing training, no staying in your comfort zone anymore. You have decided the result you want and now you are building it. You're not trying, you are doing it. There are no 'if's' or 'but's', no plan B's – nothing that distracts from Plan A, the only one you need to succeed.

A long while ago, a great warrior faced a situation which made it necessary for him to make a decision to ensure him success on the battlefield. He was about to send his armies against a powerful foe, whose men outnumbered his own. He loaded his soldiers into boats, sailed to the enemy's country, unloaded soldiers and equipment, then gave the order to burn the ships that carried them. Addressing his men before the first battle, he said, "You see the boats going up in smoke. That means we cannot leave these shores alive unless we win! We now have no choice – *we win or we perish!* They Won.

That is the level of confidence you need to have in yourself. I can assure you, if you attack your goals with the same level of confidence and determination to win shown in this story, you will succeed.

And that is how you build a great body. Remember, it's not about the plan or the diet, its about your focus, if you decide what you are going to do and make it the only logical option, then that's it, isn't it? Someone can offer you ice cream, you can see a good late night film and that could disrupt your sleep and make you too tired for tomorrow's workout, but they aren't options, right? You want to win right? Eating ice cream is not part of winning, so it doesn't happen; don't think, "that looks really good, and I have trained hard today." Think instead… I want to win, that is losing, that is not part of success, I want a great body, not an ice cream, it becomes a no-contest. Remember you're going to do it, in fact it's already done, you're just waiting for your body to realize what you've done. If you know nothing is going to stop you, your body might as well change now!

You might think you don't need to get focused and do any of this, but if you don't, then you will always be waiting for tomorrow before you start anything, and tomorrow never comes. Just remember you always have the power to be your own hero, to look, feel and perform how you want to, but first you need to zone in on what that is and then do it.

Once you start doing that, things with just keep building and building, you will never stop. You might wonder how success is made – it's made by habit, the habit of always doing your best and never giving up. Now you know, its time to build your success and get the body you want.

Finally, to make sure you stick with your plans, although focus is the number one thing you need, there are a few other ways to make yourself more focused and really stay on track, and that's to hold yourself accountable for everything you do. For example, make bets with friends about your goals, take pictures of yourself and put them on social networks and write about your new goal, then you have to achieve it – and take pictures of your food, so if you eat bad or good, you really know about it – and now its not just about winning, but also not losing!

Part Two!

This is the start of how to get you that great body. Wouldn't you like it if there was a simple and effective way to stay healthy and lean all year round, have loads of energy and not need to count calories, weigh food or do any other stuff like that? Wouldn't it be brilliant if you could live by one simple rule to make eating easier and more effective?

Well, it just so happens there is, and it has been used for millions of years by every human being up until just a few hundred years ago. It is clean unprocessed foods; yes, that's it. You probably think it can't be that simple, but think about it, 200 years ago we had pretty much no obesity, we were fitter and stronger. Visit a tribe untouched by civilization and you will notice no one is overweight and unhealthy, and its simply because they don't eat anything unnatural.

It's a simple approach, but it stood the test of time – nothing processed. It either grows in the ground or has a face; that is where your food should come from, the less it has done to it, the better it will be for your body.

You see, we are meant to eat natural real foods, I don't think anyone can argue with this fact. We are not meant to eat endless unnatural and processed sugars or grains, we are designed to thrive on clean foods; not survive on sugars and junk food and just about get through the day.

You see all processed foods do one simple thing to the body; they increase the burden, basically slowing it down. Its like when you load you car up with more stuff, it doesn't drive as well and just isn't at responsive, the human body is no different.

I call it the total body burden. Basically it means the more stresses you put on the body, the worse it will work, from fat burning to concentration, and the wrong food can be a big burden. If we evolved and developed on unprocessed, wholesome totally organic foods, then why would we stop eating them? They are obviously the perfect fuel for us, which we ate for millions of years. We were not fat then, had more energy and in most cases, were healthier. We did not evolve on sugars, caffeine, alcohol or anything else like this.

Putting that stuff in your body and expecting a good result is like putting diesel into a petrol car - bad news!

But, when you start removing these toxic foods, suddenly the body starts to work in a much better way; energy levels come back up, health improves and body-fat drops rapidly because you have reduced the burden on your body. You've let the brakes off. Instead of your body struggling to survive on the wrong fuel, it starts to thrive on the right one – clean unprocessed foods.

So my challenge to you is to try 14 days of clean eating and focusing on what you really want, and watch your body-fat reduce and things change.

To do this there are a few foods you need to remove:

All processed foods, this includes cakes, pastry, chocolate, all junk food and microwave meals. Basically, eating these foods no matter how low in calories won't do you any good because the foods are totally devoid of any nutrients such as vitamins or minerals and are normally just loaded with sugars or hydrogenated fats, both of which will have no beneficial effects for changing the way you look.

All wheat and gluten products need to be removed, this includes all breads, pasta, biscuits, anything with wheat in it. Of course, these foods are removed for a multitude of reasons, the biggest one is that most people struggle to digest a protein in wheat found in the gluten known as Glaidin. This ends up making the average person feeling bloated, tired and fatigued, not exactly how you want to feel when you're trying to exercise to build a better body.

All sugar – this shouldn't really need any explaining, everyone knows sugar is pretty much a toxin, its extremely unnatural, and without going into too much detail, rapidly spikes insulin (the fat storage hormone) and is stored as fat extremely fast, this is just a one of the reasons to cut sugar out, do it now and you will feel a lot better very fast.

Pasteurized and homogenized dairy – I'm not saying you should not have dairy products *per se*, but most commercial dairy as it gets heavily processed and is totally different from the raw form you find coming straight from the cow. The lactose in dairy is also very hard to digest and we generally lose the ability to digest lactose after we stop breast-feeding. This leaves the body unable to digest the dairy products, then because of this, we actually have to engulf the lactose with large amounts of mucus, this often gives people the sensation of having either an allergy or just feeling very tired and with stomach pains – from the body trying to break down the lactose found in dairy.

You are probably wondering what is left to eat. Well, there are loads of things, just think of it this way, if it grows in the ground, or has a face, you can eat it, from chicken to beef or pineapples to rice, but focus on more fresh vegetables, fruits, plenty of high quality organic meat, fish, eggs and some natural unprocessed whole grains such as quinoa, brown rice, etc.

That is the basics of it, remove those three foods and you will soon be feeling better than you ever have. Of course, if you are trying to get really lean and look better than you ever have, I'm afraid to say just eating less-processed foods is not going to solve everything. If you do just want to lose some body-fat and get to a healthy weight, just doing the above should work fine. However, just from the fact you are reading this book, I'm guessing you're not interested in just looking good, you want to look great – so here are a few tips to help you look better than ever.

The first is to eat 3 meals a day and try to avoid snacking, I know this is totally contrary to everything you read in most magazines, but don't worry, I'm just ahead of the game and everyone else is just behind. You see, if the read the studies, they'd show you the obvious fact that you want to burn body-fat when you're not exercising, which is most of the time, and you need to eat no more often that every 4-5 hours. The reason for this is because when you don't eat for around 5 hours or so, you actually allow the liver to deplete its normal stores of sugar and lower insulin levels. Then, after this point, you start to burn stored body-fat as fuel. If you eat every 3 hours, you actually are always using your liver to breakdown the foods you have just eaten, and either use them or store them as fat, there is actually very little time when you are using your own body-fat stores as fuel.

You see, the more often you eat, the more you spike insulin levels – the hormone which tells your body to shut off fat-burning and start fat-storing, so even a small snack late at night or any other time will actually decrease fat burning and start increasing fat storage.

Basically, if you eat 3 times a day and avoid snacking, you will actually be burning more body-fat as energy than if you ate every 3 hours. Don't worry about the stories that if you eat less than every 3 hours your metabolism will slow down. They are simply not true, it actually takes about 5-8 hours for an average-sized meal to fully digest, so if you eat anymore often than this, you are just putting food you eat on top of food you're digesting.

And that's it, getting in shape is easier than you think. Get focused and decide what you want, then stop eating processed foods, and focus on just having 3 meals a day to help increase fat burning, and you will be well on your way towards getting in the best shape of your life.

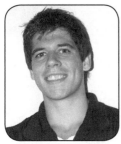

About Oliver

Oliver Chapman is the owner of Renaissance Fitness and is a body transformation expert, focusing on helping people to achieve results they never thought possible. His passion is helping people to become their own hero by making people look, feel and perform at their very best.

This is done through his very successful Personal Training business, where he uses many different methods to help people from all walks of life to achieve more than they ever thought possible.

Although he is only 21 years old, he has studied with some of the world's top experts in health and fitness, and reads between 50 and 100 books a year to further his knowledge, and is establishing himself as the 'go to' person for body transformation training and rapid fat-loss. He has been weight training and exercising since his early teenage years. He has developed a huge passion for helping people achieve their goals from the knowledge he has gained from studying with various experts, and through his own trial-and-error from years of walking his talk and constantly challenging himself in every area of life, from sky dives and weightlifting competitions to the development of his own Personal Training business.

He embraces the idea that fitness and health is not just about looking good, but also using it to help develop a strong mind and healthy body, and challenging yourself inside and outside of the gym to achieve more than just great fitness, but also because improving health and getting the body you want should help you live the life you want to live, by having more confidence in the way you look, feel and perform to help take on any challenges life throws at you.

He realizes that the way you look, feel and perform should be part of a holistic approach to improving every other area of your life, which is built into his Personal Training and almost certainly one reason why he is able to get such ground-breaking results with his Personal Training clients.

To learn more about Oliver and what he does, go to his website: www.olliechapman.com

CHAPTER 9

Be Fit For Life

By Damien Maher

If you are reading this book, you are probably pretty serious about your health. You want to get into better shape, lose some weight, and get some focus in your fitness.

Or you might be a coach or personal trainer who is looking for some help in getting the best results from your clients.

Either way, you are willing to invest a bit of money in return for some knowledge that will get you closer to the perfect you. You have probably bought other information products, books, pills and potions all claiming to have the secret to weight loss and the perfect body.

But has any of it worked? Are you in the best shape of your life? Do you wake up every morning happy in the knowledge that whatever clothes you put on will look great? Are your clients walking billboards for your business? Are they stopped on the street and asked how they stay in such good shape?

If so, you can save yourself some time and stop reading now because you already know what I know. If not, read on because you have finally invested in a product that will actually get you closer to your goal, because in this chapter I am offering proof of a formula that works.

I am going to share with you the story of just one of my clients that has achieved their dream body. And not just for a fleeting moment. Pauline, an ordinary working mother like you or one of your clients, lost an amazing 126 lbs in 12 months. And even more amazingly, she has defied the statistics and kept that weight off now for four years and counting. In fact, every year, Pauline's body gets better as she continues on the path to which I guided her in 2007.

As coaches, personal trainers or gym instructors, we have the opportunity to act as a catalyst in the transformation of someone else's life. Clients originally come to us with the goal of losing weight, toning up and getting fitter, but the reality is that we will have more contact time with our clients than doctors, and so we will have a bigger opportunity to influence their health than many other professions.

Misinformed and misguided, they have trudged through a minefield of diets, infomercials and marketing all designed to stimulate faith and hope that they might have found the Holy Grail for weight loss. They go on a journey similar to a carousel at a fairground, going around in circles, up and down, before coming back to the same spot. It is the story for so many attempting to lose weight. They inevitably end up back in the same spot — having lost time, energy and finances as they enthusiastically went nowhere.

Brian Tracy, one of the world's leading experts on success psychology and personal achievement, has identified two new 'diseases' rampant in developed countries. These diseases could be applied to the fitness industry, as there are many people afflicted with the symptoms associated with these diseases. These are the 'something-for-nothing' disease and the 'quick-fix' disease. Those suffering from 'something-for-nothing' want weight loss without dieting, fitness without exercise, and perfect health while eating and drinking whatever they want.

Those with 'quick-fix' disease want to take a pill, go to sleep, and wake up skinny. They are suckers for the latest miracle solution and buy fat-burning creams, which never yield the results they crave. But with a little perseverance and a better work ethic, they could easily reach their goals. The very act of seeking a 'quick fix' or wanting 'something for nothing' is weak. But setting a worthy goal for something you want and reaching it through determination and hard work changes the very fibre of your being and makes you strong - physically, mentally and emotionally. George Bernard Shaw said, "Doing what needs to be done may not make you happy, but it will make you great."

The reason most people don't lose weight is because they don't care about it enough. People who care take action. They are committed to accomplishing what they set out to do. They don't do the least to get the most, they do whatever it takes. Most people say they are doing the best they can. Stop. The question is, are they doing whatever it takes? To achieve long-term weight loss, you need to work towards mastery. Mastery is a product of consistently going beyond your limits.

Every journey is accompanied by risks, and your first challenge is to find a trainer/coach that will flash the light along the path they want you to follow.

It is hard for someone to go through a weight-loss journey on their own, and in this tech-driven world there are plenty of places for people to turn to for help. They search the Internet to guide them on their journey, but it is hard for them to be able to distinguish between a coach who can deliver on the bravado. They are not doing the jobs that they claim to have done.

Choosing a personal trainer or coach is like drilling for oil - it's fraught with risk. No one in his or her right mind would simply go out in their backyard and start digging with the hope of hitting a 'gusher'. The same can be said of walking into a gym hoping to find the right trainer for you. Oil companies invest their time and do extensive research to analyse seismic and geological maps. They take samples of rocks and soils, study fault lines, and look at the surrounding area to see if there are other formations that would justify 'poking' a hole in the ground.

They compare all this and decide that if everything looks favourable, only then will the company proceed to drill for oil. That is how your search for a trainer should begin. You should do extensive research into finding your coach or mentor, because it is like any relationship. A long-term romantic liaison does not begin by walking into a random bar and having a 'lucky dip' with the available clientele before embarking on a relationship that could change your life. That may happen in fairy tales, but the reality of finding a suitable partner or your personal trainer is entirely different.

The people who are the best in the world at anything — whether at swimming, golf, ballet or business — all studied and apprenticed under someone who was a master, to learn the critical skills and tools to become better at their craft. Masters allowed them to do the right things first time, and simultaneously avoided making the most basic and stupid mistakes. It's the mistakes and setbacks that keep people frustrated and unhappy in their quest to lose weight or improve health. Just about the time you are starting to climb out of the last hole you dug, you promptly start digging another.

So if you are looking to lose weight, you should find a mentor who never stops studying. If you are a coach, never stop learning and seek out those who know more than you. The best in the world know they must practice to improve on a daily basis if they are to retain their greatness.

All the hard work in the world won't bring you to your weight-loss goal if you are not doing the right things. I had many clients come to me who worked out five times a week and were disciplined with their food, but got no results.

Why? Because they were relying on bits and pieces of information they picked up here and there. They had no master to guide them. All their hard work was for nothing. When they reapplied that energy and focus under my guidance, the results astounded even them.

Yes, weight-loss success will be a result of your hard work and a positive mental attitude, but most important of all, it will be your training and nutrition program. Every person at the top of their game in golf surrounds themselves with coaches who can, in their case, watch their swing.

They have the exact same problem you and I do — they can't see themselves when they swing their golf clubs. So they surround themselves with people who watch — who can coach them on where they going wrong as needed.

But not everyone goes the road of coaching for weight loss. When they are sick, they go to a doctor; when their car breaks down, they take it to a mechanic. But when someone gains weight or is overweight with existing health conditions, why don't they go to trainers?

Some people are embarrassed and they want to get themselves in shape before contacting a trainer. That's completely nuts as any good trainer or coach has a gym with people of all shapes and sizes as they progress through the stages on the journey to fitness. People in gyms that work, who train with coaches that are serious, have clients that support each other and revel in each new client that comes along; so if you take that step, you are immediately among friends.

Some people who want to lose weight and get into shape say they can't afford a trainer. They think that is just for Hollywood stars or really wealthy people. The question I ask them is: how much money have your fitness and nutrition mistakes cost you throughout your life? Not to mention how much anger and frustration have you left in the gym and at home, as you didn't know how to achieve and sustain weight loss? Invest in yourself. As they say, you're worth it.

And if you decide to work through your excuses and stop relying on trial and error, permanent change is possible. It is achievable. And it happened to an ordinary working mother who decided that she was sick and tired of being sick and tired. She threw off her embarrassment, discarded her excuses and said, "Right. I have got to do something about this or I will be a fat woman for the rest of my life." She wanted change and she was willing to do whatever it took. All she needed was someone to guide her hard work and direct her focus in the right direction.

Pauline Fitzsimons contacted me via email on the 26th January 2007 with the following email.

"Hi Damien,
I noticed your poster at the gym and I had a look at your website. I am not really sure if your expertise extends to my issues, but I thought I would reach out and see what you think. I am 40 years old and obese (BMI 38) and have recently started to exercise for the first time in years. While I have lost some weight, progress is slow and I am not sure if even what I am doing is the right thing. My 2007 goal is to become fit and lose some weight, but I know I need some help.
Best Regards, Pauline"

My initial venture into marketing my services was a poster on the wall of a large health club chain, a Big Box gym. I had used social proof of clients on my website as a means of marketing, but when Pauline viewed these pictures she could not relate to them. She would have been happy with their 'before' photos, never mind they're 'after,' but still it encouraged Pauline to make contact with me.

We arranged to meet for a conversation to see if we made a good fit for each other. An initial meeting is very important for both the trainer and the client to ensure they are singing from the same hymn sheet.

A client looking to lose over 100 lbs will be embarking on a long- term relationship, so it is important that both parties know what is expected of each other. Prior to our meeting, I had sent Pauline an initial questionnaire where she could clarify her goals and her expectations.

In addition to this, I asked Pauline to complete a food diary where she would record her food, the times she ate, liquids she drank (water, with caffeine, alcohol, etc.), sleep, exercise and relaxation habits for the week.

It is said that the shortest of pencils is better than the longest of memories, and a food diary enlightens you and your coach to your eating habits, and why you may not be making progress in your body-shaping program. It also gave me an idea of where Pauline currently was in terms of meal frequency, portion sizes and where I thought we could start her program.

Keeping track of what you eat is one of the easiest secrets to fat-loss success I can think of. If it makes you think twice about what you are consuming, then it is worth it. Georgia University conducted a study looking at the effects of eating one meal a day with a total caloric intake equal to the other test subjects eating six smaller meals a day.

The one meal a day group's body went into fat-storing mode, as the body was unable to break down the excess calories. The other group kept fuelling the flames of metabolism by eating little and often. It should be noted that Sumo Wrestlers skip breakfast and eat one meal a day with a massive caloric intake. By eating regularly you will be controlling your blood sugar levels much better, hence this can reduce your sweet cravings.

The completion of the food diary also gave me an indication of how compliant Pauline was going to be. The food diary is one of the keys to uncovering your weight-loss roadblocks.

You can either take the time to write out your diary or you can make excuses and say you remember it, but oral food diaries are not worth the paper they are printed on. If you cannot understand where your problems lie, you need to reach out for someone who can help you. When you have to present your food diary for inspection to a peer or your personal trainer, you will be less likely to be caught with your hand in the cookie jar and you may just achieve the results that your training deserves.

During our initial meeting, Pauline started to share her story with me. Pauline was the classic working Mum, with a demanding job and two young children to deal with.

When she wasn't working, she was trying to make it up to the kids because of the guilt that every working Mum feels, so making some personal time wasn't an option in her mind's eye. A routine health screening at work brought to light that she was beginning to develop serious health problems: high cholesterol with the prospect of diabetes, and with high blood pressure on the way if she did not take corrective action. I made her realize that in fact neglecting her personal welfare was indeed being Selfish to her kids, and not Selfless as she had tried to convince me.

The road to redemption did not start immediately. She knew she needed help but was unsure where to start. After years of trying and failing the 'Quick Fix' diets, she knew the only way to go was healthy eating and exercise, but she wasn't sure she had the nerve to face the gym, thinking surely that's where all the slim people go.

So she had started to swim 4 times a week and eat a little better, after 3 months she had lost 7 lbs and realised quickly that at this rate of progress, she was unlikely to ever succeed.

Her good friends Frank and Julie had recommended she should try a Personal Trainer, and she had noticed my poster up in the gym, so she decided first to mail me and see as a trainer if I dealt with obesity.

I assured Pauline that anyone could succeed if they just follow the directions I give them and add hard work and commitment. Famed Green Bay Packer Coach Vince Lombardi said it best when he said "the only time success comes before work is in the dictionary."

There is no glamour or magic associated with hard work. I explained the difference between horizontal and vertical time lines. Long-term weight loss responds better to consistent actions done over time. This would be represented on a horizontal timeline axis. You don't become overweight overnight and you will not become slim tomorrow from five hours of activity today.

So the questions were not so much about how she will win the game of weight loss, but more how she was going to play the second half of the game. We looked at setting long-term and short-term goals, but more importantly we looked at what were the behaviours that would need to happen to make those goals a reality.

Goals act as lighthouses to keep you focused when the seas become rough. Losing nine stone seems like a daunting prospect similar to chopping down a big Oak tree. You stand back at the tree and say I will never chop that tree down, but by making a plan we had attempted to sharpen our blade, and if we took a few swings of the axe everyday, eventually the tree would fall down.

We took measurements that we would regularly check so we could ensure that we were on track with our goal. Before photos, front, side and back gave us visual information, circumference measurements would measure the inches lost and a body fat % was measured using 12 sites with a Harpendon John Bull calipers. Body fat was taken consistently on the same day, same time every week for consistency.

During our first month of training, I asked Pauline how she felt her body was progressing. "I guess the first month is always the hardest. I had never done any weight training before in my life, and aside from a couple lengths of breaststroke, my cardio levels were not up too much.

So I started my weight training on 17th February. While I was unable to walk the next day after the experience, it was not as bad as I expected." Pauline performed a weights-based exercise program alternating between upper and lower body to increase peripheral heart flow.

Quads exercises like squats/split squats were alternated with lat pull-downs. The following pairing would see hamstring exercises paired with shoulder exercises to make the heart push blood the longest distance upstairs and downstairs to these muscles.

It is this style of training sometimes referred to as German Body Composition training popularized by strength coach Charles Poliquin that changes the pH of your blood encouraging your body to produce more lactate, releasing growth hormone to build muscle.

More muscle or lean body mass means you have a bigger engine to burn more fuel and hence over time faster fat loss. Short rest intervals of between 30-60 seconds increase production of lactate, which leads to dramatic increases in growth hormone in your body, enabling it to build muscle to burn fat and lose weight.

This method leads to dramatic fat loss and is effective in developing strength endurance. One pound of fat needs nine calories a day to be maintained while one pound of muscle needs 50 calories a day to be maintained. Our goal was to increase your engine size, which burns off more calories.

Female clients can gain 10-12 lbs of muscle in exchange for 10-12 lbs of fat in two months. This is equal to burning off 500 calories a day, which is equivalent to a pound of fat lost each week. It is not during training that you burn the majority of calories, but it is post-exercise and this is why strength training and interval training are superior methods for fat loss over aerobic training.

If it didn't burn, make her feel short of breath and even make her feel nauseous in the first 20 minutes, it would not work for Pauline nor would it work for you. You are either not working hard enough, or taking too long on your rest periods if you do not experience these feelings.

The time under tension (when the muscle is working) should be between 40 and 120 seconds worth of work per exercise set. If you choose the correct weight, the muscle will tremble on the last few repetitions, but it will ultimately change shape.

Pauline's initial squat was her bodyweight with the assistance of holding onto a machine. A bodyweight squat to squash your calves means that you lift 75% of your body weight and if you are overweight this increases the effort you must make. So even when she performed bodyweight squats, it was the equivalent of 90-100kg on your first day. My role as coach was to ensure that everything was set up for Pauline and to make sure she focused on the exercises she was trying to perform.

It is a daunting experience for someone to walk into a new gym with a goal of losing weight. Pauline seemed undeterred but said she was too busy sweating and concentrating to notice if anyone else was watching, or laughing at her in the gym!!!

For the next few weeks, Pauline completed the weight circuit twice a week with me, and I gradually showed her how to use the equipment and fill in her own program as she gained the confidence to go up to the weights room on her own.

In this time, I also did some interval training on the treadmill and made one critical change to her diet; recommending protein and raw nuts for breakfast. Protein is derived from the Greek word of primary importance, and it helps detoxify the liver, repair the immune system, provides satiety and it creates a thermogenic effect to burn energy just through digesting the protein you are eating.

One of the most important functions of protein is that it contains nitrogen – which repairs the muscles that would have been damaged from exercise. Protein increases the release of the neuro-transmitter Dopamine with has been linked with increasing neural drive. The raw nuts provided fats that would help balance her blood sugar and reduce her food cravings. Nuts increase the release of the neurotransmitter acetyl choline which has been linked with improving decision-making. The main supplement I gave during this time to Pauline was large dosages of fish oil.

Julia Ross, in her book the Diet Cure, talks of treating Irish alcoholics with fish oil to reduce their cravings. Alcohol, when used in conjunction with medicinal cough syrups, helps get the medicine into the blood stream quicker by acting like a sugar. By applying the same principle to weight-loss clients, it reduces sweet cravings. It has been used in incidences of depression, which often leads to comfort eating. It improves your mood by helping your body increase the production of the neurotransmitter serotonin, which makes you happy.

Fish oil turns on fat-burning lipolytic cells and it turns off fat-storing lipogenic cells and it increases the permeability of our cells, so we can get energy into them instead of depositing it into our ever-willing fat cells. Fat cells are the hardest working cells in your body, and they never take days off.

There is a rule when you are implementing changes in your habits. It is called the Magic Rule of 21, and it says that it takes 21 days in a row of performing a new behaviour in order to crystallise that new behaviour into a habit.

One important habit we set into motion was that we had set days and times for training — to ensure that training would become second nature and a way of life for Pauline.

Many times I see trainers overwhelm their clients with information. The trainers are trying to help and share their wisdom but it often frightens the clients. I often explain it by the story of how chefs cook frogs. If a chef drops a frog into boiling water the frog will hit the water and his reflexes will immediately get him to jump out of the water.

A better way to cook the frog would be to place him in a pot of luke-warm water where he is comfortable and gradually increase the temperature until he passes out. So after one month, Pauline had three good new habits. She trained three times per week, ate a good breakfast every day that would balance out her blood sugar, and she took fish oil to turn on her fat-burning cells and reduce her fat-storing cells.

When working with overweight people, the initial weight loss is slow. Pauline's initial weight loss averaged at only 1 lb per week as she built up her habits. It is very common for someone changing a nutrition program to start absorbing nutrients for the first time in a long time and this may increase lean body mass. They have been previously malnourished with a diet lacking in nutrients. That is why there might be inches lost, but not so much weight on the scale, so it is important not to become too disheartened. You are merely building a bigger engine to burn more calories.

By the second month, Pauline was confident to go up to the gym and complete her program on her own. She still found it difficult but she was determined to persist. I continued to work with her on her diet, replacing refined processed food with fresh meat, fish, salad, vegetables and fruit, eliminating soda and alcohol and increasing the quantity of water.

Lunch was fish or meats with salads, and dinners were meat and fish and vegetables. Pauline benefited from a diet that was higher in proteins and healthy fats, and by cycling carbohydrates in and out of her diet during the week to speed up her metabolism, and to prevent muscle lost by replenishing the glycogen or energy in her muscles.

She still received personal training once a week, and in her words "these were always the hardest sessions." I pushed her really hard and ensured she performed to the maximum of her ability, never letting her stand still as I knew what she could achieve. Each week I measured her body fat percentage, and reviewed her food diary for the week — to make sure she stayed on track and to chart her progress.

Near the end of March, I changed her program. A program is only as good as the time it takes you to adapt to it and it took Pauline out of her comfort zone as she had become familiar and comfortable with the old program, and so was her body, so it was time for a change.

People she knew had started to notice the changes in her and she felt so much better. The first big challenge Pauline faced was when she was due to go on holidays to Florida for two weeks. I designed a program she could complete in the villa without any weights. Her perception was that this would be so much easier. But by manipulating the exercise variables in her training program like repetitions, sets, tempo or speed of exercises, rest periods or order of exercises, she was unable to sit comfortably on the flight to Orlando as her rear end and legs hurt so much!

One of the principles of training is progressive overload. It is essential if your goal is long-term fat loss. The best way to analyse your program in the gym is that each time you go, you should be 2% stronger. This could equate to a weight 2% heavier for the same number of reps or the same weight lifted for an additional repetition.

This was a key turning point for Pauline in her belief in what she could achieve. She felt she didn't do brilliantly, but she came home 4 lbs lighter and she had worked out 5 times. She arrived home on Saturday into Dublin and got straight back up to the gym on Sunday. By mid April, her weight loss had speeded up as new habits were integrated with old habits to help her lose over 2 stone or 28 lbs and her energy levels were so much higher.

During the second month, Pauline had been very anxious about her food and found it quite difficult to manage if she had to eat out. She often left long gaps between meals until she got home and could cook for herself. Eating out for every meal except breakfast for 2 whole weeks taught her how to make the best food choices from any menu, and how to mix and match menu items so she always had enough of the right foods to eat.

In the third month of her training program, Pauline now had 2 new programs that she alternated between each time she trained. It added a variety to the training and at this stage, I also increased the workload of her training frequency. She now weight-trained 4 times per week with 1 cardio session on the treadmill when she could fit it in.

To recover from holidays, I asked Pauline to follow a stricter diet for 2 weeks - a diet Bootcamp.

By mid May, she was 3 stone or 42 lbs down and still feeling great. Julie and Frank, the initial catalysts that advised her to hire a trainer came back from their travels and were amazed by the changes in her. She did have a bottle of champagne to celebrate with them; she was very happy with what she had achieved, but even happier as she was now 100% confident that she could achieve her final target. She didn't have a drink since. She hasn't decided to be a non-drinker, but she said she would wait till her birthday before making a decision. In Ireland, believe me, this is a big deal. Most social occasions involve alcohol and people who don't drink alcohol are uncommon.

The months were rolling on, and during her fourth month, things got a lot easier, as her newfound good habits became engraved on her lifestyle. She now trains 4 to 5 times per week, and she eats a healthy diet. Friends no longer comment when she refuses the offer of a drink.

To add variety to her cardio, I consistently changed the format and introduced boxing and rowing interval training, in addition to introducing 2 new weight-training programs every 3 weeks. Pauline enjoyed the boxing and she now rows with a buddy once a week at work, which motivates her to do that.

She found the weight training enjoyable, admittedly she found it tough at the time, but then she feels so great afterwards. Motivation is easier when you are getting the results you want to keep you on target. When you think back to last February and she could barely squat, she needed support to stand back up; now she can regularly do full squats with it and can do it with 50 kg on her back — though she was herself 90 lbs lighter to prove it!

Four years later, Pauline still trains four times a week and follows the nutritional guidelines I set her. As I learn new methods and facts that promote health, so does Pauline. It is important to remain challenged and constantly surprise your body with your training programs because fitness is a lifestyle. People ask me 'What will happen after I have lost the weight and I stop the training?' I reply, "Why would you stop?"

Exercise and nutritional changes are healthy lifestyle choices, and the choices you make can help you Be Fit For Life. Is it hard work? Well the answer to that is yes, but then a lot of the worthwhile things you achieve in life are hard work.

The ability to work hard is in all of us, what you need to do is get your priorities right. Examine your life and look at the obstacles that are preventing you from opting for a healthier lifestyle, resolve these issues and most of all believe in yourself. The ability to be successful is in us all.

Pauline started out on this journey because of health concerns. Looking great has been a wonderful bonus, but whatever the motivation, the most wonderful thing is how much energy she has now. As she approached her 45th birthday, she looks and feels better now than she did in her 20s, so she plans to put into practice that life truly begins in your 40s and it is never too late to change!!!

Every journey needs a guide, and as a coach I am delighted I could play a part in Pauline's journey. She made a decision and she empowered herself to regain control of her health. Areas of your life that you are not in power over like your health, someone else will 'overpower,' like a doctor, because they do not believe that you can do it for yourself.

But success leaves clues. If you want to go on a similar journey, follow the trail that someone who has worn those shoes has left behind. This can shorten the journey and you can learn from their mistakes so you do not have to repeat them.

The only thing you need to do is to take action and to take the first step. It is the journey of a thousand miles or the loss of 9 stone in 12 months that began with a single step. You will be amazed by what you can achieve.

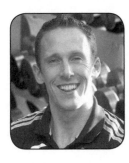

About Damien

Damien Maher is a strength and conditioning specialist from Sandyford, Dublin. His company, Be Fit For Life Performance Centre Ltd is housed in a 3,000 sq ft personal training gym - which has helped hundreds of clients of all ages and from all walks of life to transform their body shapes, increase their energy levels and adopt a healthier lifestyle.

Damien's method is the result of his personal experience as a former professional soccer player, combined with the advanced theories of European sports science and the principles of modern strength and conditioning systems.

He travels extensively to learn from the world's leading experts in strength training, nutrition, functional medicine, supplementation, treatment and the rehabilitation of injuries.

He uses this knowledge and his own vast experience to develop training programs that help each individual client achieve their specific goals for which he guarantees results.

Damien was the Fitness Expert on TV3's reality TV show Inside & Out, and he writes a weekly column in the health supplement of the Irish Independent.

The success stories on his website: www.befitforlife.ie are a testimony to Damien's vision, hard work and dedication to his clients.

CHAPTER 10

Goal Setting, Action Planning, and Achievement

By Nick Berry

Anyone who has done any amount of personal growth research, specifically in the goal setting category, has probably heard this story. I believe it was a class of Harvard graduates, in the 70's or early 80's. The entire class was surveyed upon graduation, and one of the questions was, "Have you set clear, written goals for your future and made plans to accomplish them?" The results of the survey were that three percent of the graduates had written goals and plans; 13 percent had goals, but they were not in writing; and 84 percent had no specific goals at all.

The story skips ahead ten years, where the members of the class were interviewed again, and the findings were incredible. The 13 percent of the class who had goals but they were not written, were earning on average twice as much as the 84 percent with no goals at all. What was more impressive was that the three percent who had clearly written goals were earning, on average, ten times as much as the other 97 percent put together.

I'm not sure that I could take this to mean that setting goals guarantees you will make more money, or writing goals out makes you more likely to achieve them. I do think it is very clear however, that having goals is a clearly superior plan to not having them. Such a substantial success rate doesn't happen by accident. If you want to achieve, you must identify goals and work with them in mind. Be it business, fitness, achievements, athletic accomplishments – it makes no difference. You are much more likely to reach your potential if you set clear goals.

When trying to undertake a particularly challenging task, it is useful to look elsewhere for analogies to help guide your actions and give you perspective. Since my background is in the fitness industry and my company, Fitness Consulting Group, works with fitness business entrepreneurs every single day, I can see firsthand the similarities between running a large organization and setting and reaching fitness goals.

What you should also be aware of is that even though I am primarily discussing fitness goals here, do not limit yourself to only fitness goals should you decide to put this into practice. The type of goal setting I will be covering can apply to every facet of your life.

First things first, and that is that it is important to have direction. If you do not take the time to determine your goals and commit to regular measurement and review, you will simply be wasting time, energy, and effort.

SPECIFIC	What exactly do I want to accomplish and why? What criteria will I be required to meet in order to reach this goal?
MEASURABLE	What are those concrete criteria? In fitness, you can measure body fat, circumference of various body parts, dress size, weight, and training performance, to name just a few
ATTAINABLE	Not to be confused with easy, attainable goals are simply not extreme. For example, your goal cannot mention that you want to be taller or look like another person. However, it should be able to be achieved realistically if broken down into smaller action steps.
RELEVANT	Is this really the goal you want to reach? Does it matter to you?
TIMELY	The goal has a deadline.

Goal setting is a process in itself, and like many things, there are good kinds and bad kinds. A bad goal is ambiguous and does not hold its maker accountable in any way. A good goal, on the other hand, is S.M.A.R.T.

Now there are many types of fitness goals, big and small, long-term and short-term, habit-based and physique-based, etc. The very first goal you should make, however, is your end goal or your big goal. In other words, start at the finish line.

As Lewis Carroll once said, "If you don't know where you are going, any road will get you there."

Before I have you write out your end goal, however, consider the following keys to writing an effective goal:

I. Write it as a positive, present-tense statement. Set a goal for what you want, not for what you don't want. Your mind can lock onto a clearly defined goal only if the goal is defined positively. Phrase your goals as if you have already achieved it. For example, instead of saying, "I will get down to 12% body fat by the first day of next year," phrase it in the present tense: "It is January 1st, and I am at 12% body fat." Avoid watered down words like "probably," "should," "could," "would," "might," or "may" when forming your goals.

II. Begin your goal statement with an "Outcome Verb." Outcome verbs such as "build, achieve, earn, grow, create" give life to your goals. Instead of saying: "I hope to lose 20 pounds," say, "I've lost 20 pounds."

III. Write goals that will have multiple steps as projects. Projects will contain small actions you can take step by step. For example, completing a 12-week workout program is a multiple-step project, while performing 5 sets of 5 reps of a particular exercise is an action step within that project.

IV. Create your goals based on your numbers. Tracking your numbers and basing your goals off current numbers will allow you to more easily see success and create the action steps necessary to achieve your goal.

So, using the criteria above, write out a S.M.A.R.T. end goal that answers the following question: In terms of your fitness, where do you want to be one year from today?

In fitness, there are primarily two types of projects that need to be considered for you to achieve the results you are looking for, exercise projects and nutrition projects.

Let's cover exercise first. Exercise really boils down to two things, a quality training program and your ability to follow that training program. Let's say your goal is to reach 12% body fat in one year. In order to reach that goal, you are likely going to have to, at a minimum, put on muscle and lose fat. In addition, improving your strength, power, and athleticism would probably be compatible with that big goal as well.

These smaller goals of gaining muscle, losing fat, increasing strength, etc. will form the "projects" that together make up the big goal. Each of these projects should be put into their own 4-12 week exercise phases. For example, you might decide that you should break down your program into four, 3-month training phases. The first phase would be geared towards general preparation. The next phase would be for strength. The third would be for muscle building, and the final would be for fat burning.

Whether this breakdown is ideal for you is not the point. The point, rather, is to be able to break down your big goal into these projects and then to break down each of these projects into even smaller action steps. Let's continue with the example I provided.

You have your big goal, and now you have your projects. What you want to do next is craft your workouts for the first project, or in this case, the general preparation phase. Putting together your workout sheet will take care of both writing out the small action steps that you need to take and giving you the means to track whether you are actually completing these steps.

The following items should go into your workout sheet:

1. The different workouts that comprise the phase. How many different workouts will there be? Will you have an "A" workout and a "B" workout that you alternate?

2. The actual exercises that are a part of each workout. Are you trying to do full body workouts? Do you have an upper body workout and a lower body workout? In what order do you perform the exercises? Do you have alternating exercises or a circuit?

3. Your set, rep, and rest scheme. How many sets and reps are you going to perform for each exercise? How much rest will you take

between sets of exercises?

4. A place to record objective data. How much weight did you lift for a certain exercise? How many sets and reps did you actually perform versus what was written in advance on the sheet?

5. The dates and times you will perform each workout. How many days a week are you going to train, and what days and times actually fit into your schedule?

6. Notes. Do you have something you would like to measure such as your weight, body fat percentage, or arm circumference at the beginning of the phase that you can measure again at the end of the phase for comparison?

Once you have your workout sheet for the phase written up, all you need to do now is take action on the days you wrote down and committed to, follow the plan, and record your data from each workout. The goals for this phase are automatically built into your workout sheet: show up for each workout and get better, objectively, each week.

Finally, as you near the end of the first project or exercise phase, you can look over all the objective data that you have recorded, evaluate your progress, and start putting together your workout sheet for the next phase. Then all you will need to do is continue this process until the end of the year.

That takes care of your exercise projects and the action planning that goes along with them. What about nutrition? Again, it is valuable to look at your end product and then decide what steps need to be taken to get there. Nutrition can be simplified to the foods and supplements you need to ingest and the dietary habits you need to follow.

Rather than trying to do overhaul your nutrition all at once, keep in mind the length of time you have to achieve your big goal, and then set up smaller projects accordingly. For example, to reach 12% body fat, you might decide upon the following projects:

1. Consume a post-workout shake within 30 minutes of each workout

2. Take 2 fish oil capsules with each meal

3. Eat 3 meals and 2 snacks per day

4. Consume an animal protein and non-starchy vegetable at each meal

5. For 90% of meals, only include foods that are meat or fish, non-starchy vegetables, and fruit and only drink calorie-free beverages

6. For 90% of meals, only include foods that are grass-fed or free-range meats, wild fish, and non-starchy vegetables and only drink water or green tea.

Continuing with the example, you should finish your first project by the end of month one. "Consuming a post-workout shake" will then be a habit that you will continue, ideally, throughout your life. By the end of month two, you should finish your second project, and so on and so forth. Each project will serve as a short-term goal, and all you need to do is set up deadlines in which to reach them.

As is the case with your workouts, it is important to record what you are actually doing each day. That way, you will be able to see if you are following through with your action steps. In the example above, a simple daily checklist will help you determine whether you are consistent with projects 1-4. For projects 5 and 6, you will need to keep a daily food log.

To review:
Achievement simply requires that you clearly determine your one big goal, break down that goal into smaller projects, define the action steps required to complete those projects, and finally, record or measure your progress along the way.

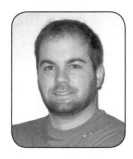

About Nick

Nick Berry has spent his entire career as an Entrepreneur in the fitness industry. His experience has given him the opportunity to become a Business Coach and Consultant, and co-owner of dozens of other businesses, which have allowed him to help thousands of other small business owners, both in and out of the fitness industry.

Nick co-founded, co-owns, and continues to build the Athletic Revolution™ and Fitness Revolution™ franchise systems. The Athletic Revolution™ (www.myathleticrevolution.com) is a youth-based sports performance franchise that began in 2009 and currently has over 30 franchise units. Fitness Revolution™ (www.fitnessrevolutionfranchise.com) is an adult fitness franchise, which began in January 2011, and currently has over 50 franchise units.

Nick partnered with Pat Rigsby in 2005 and they continue to operate Fitness Consulting Group, (www.fitbusinessinsider.com) from which they offer their fitness business consulting programs. He has helped build and co-owns the International Youth Conditioning Association, which is considered the premier international authority on youth conditioning and athletic development (www.iyca.org). He also was a co-author of the International Best Selling *Total Body Breakthroughs* book in the spring of 2011.

CHAPTER 11

Get Off The Scale To Get Results

By Holly Rigsby

How many times are you doing it? Once a week…once a day…several times a day?

Stepping on the scale – wishing, hoping, praying as you hold your breath and stare down at the number you see above your toes, almost afraid to look. Wondering why, despite your efforts to eat right and exercise, this number will not budge – or worse, only goes up!

Have you ever stopped to realize how this obsession with a number on the scale is actually holding you back from making progress?

Sure we all begin a fitness plan with the ultimate goal to drop some weight, however when it comes to the process women must go through to get results, many get caught up with the number on the scale, and end up losing sight of the most important changes that are taking place – ones that a scale simply cannot measure.

I'd like to share a story from a mom I have worked with since the start of 2011 who broke her addiction to the scale. Her story hits home for I can personally relate to the struggles she experienced as she strived to get results and achieve a fit and healthy body. Her transformation also demonstrates the potential we all have to transform, when we take the power away from the scale and begin to focus on the success that truly does matter – to true and lasting body shaping results.

I'll now turn it over to Niki.

"Never in a million years would I have ever been convinced that breaking free from the scale would allow me to drop 2 sizes and completely reshape my body.

Believe it or not.... before I began my Fit Yummy Mummy transformation, I was broken, lost and unhealthy. My journey had started, like so many other moms, after having my son. I'm embarrassed to say that I weighed a whopping 197 lbs. on the day I gave birth. At that point, I knew that it was going to be a struggle to lose the baby weight.

I ended up working on my body for 8 years! After dozens of failed attempts with fad diets, diet pills and even joining a health club...I felt like nothing was going to work for me. I would do great for a few weeks and then right after the scale started to move, I would quit – and the weight came back on.

In my eyes, nothing worked and I always failed.

I was forever searching for "the" program that was going to do it for me.... the program that was going to help me lose those stubborn pounds, because then I would be skinny.

My self-esteem was also at an all time low. I truly believed that the answer to all my life's problems at that time was held in that number that was on the scale. I became obsessed with that number, weighing progress, success and who I was, fully based on that number.

I was a slave to the scale.

I was always thinking about the pounds I wanted to lose, the size I wanted to be and the figure that I longed to have. I thought that if I could just lose that weight and be skinny that I could finally be happy, beautiful, care free, desirable. What I didn't fully understand was the underlying issue. I hated....ME.

Prior to signing up for ClubFYM in November of 2010, I had lost enough weight to reach 134 – I thought this would make me happy, but I was still round and jiggly, and I still couldn't shake a size 8.

I was doing cardio a LOT along with some workout DVDs. I'd even add in power walks several times per week! In my mind I kept thinking that all this exercise should be making me skinny!!!

I was so frustrated with "all my efforts" and my inability to lose any more weight. I thought that it was SO UNFAIR! What I didn't realize is that I didn't have a clue how to be healthy.

I had originally purchased the Fit Yummy Mummy eBook and interval soundtracks in the spring of 2010. I had gotten Holly's emails for over a year, so I finally decided to join ClubFYM in November of 2010, because something told me that I needed more. There was something missing. To me, at that point, the missing piece was weight loss. Plus I had NO intention of doing a 'challenge,' because at that point, I thought it wasn't for me at all and would be a waste of my time. And I had no time or interest in the forums.

January 2011 – it all changed.

I just knew that this year was going to be different. It was going to be amazing. I didn't know how or why. I just knew. So I decided on a total whim to join the New Year's Transformation Challenge.

Previously, I had found challenges to be silly. I now realize it was all my insecurity of actually being able to accomplish anything I set out to do. But something inside told me that I needed to give it a try this time. What was even greater was my desire to purchase the Transformation Kit, since it had everything I needed to do, laid out step-by-step.

While my goal was to lose weight and eat right, I also thought I should really work on my self-esteem.

What I went through in 12 weeks was a journey of self-discovery and healing.

In working on my external appearance, I discovered that so many of the reasons I was lacking in results, my self-worth was wrapped up in issues I needed to deal with from my past. Without even trying, I found myself reflecting and discussing my journey.

I was constantly asking myself "why?" And when I thought I had found the answer, I would go back and reflect more. This was happening while I was learning the FYM lifestyle of the right way to eat, and the best ways to workout.

By the time my 12 weeks were complete, what I found was new respect for myself!

I broke free from the scale and from the chains that had been holding me back. I was able kick my negative self-image to the curb. When I was done with the challenge, I actually saw myself through new eyes.

I saw a woman that had features she had never had before.

Confidence. Pride. Self-worth. Beauty. Love. Respect.

The biggest eye opener was that the scale barely budged. In 12 weeks, I only lost 2 pounds! However, I was able to lose 13 overall inches and dropped from a size 7/8 to a size 3/4.

Here are my 12 week results...
Weight: 130 - 128
Size: 7/8 - 3/4
Mommy Tummy: 31 - 27.5
Hips: 37.5 - 36
Thighs: 22.5 - 20.5

A size 3/4! I have NEVER been this size in my life! I remember wearing a size 7/8 in 6th grade. What I didn't realize was that looking in the mirror each day, I always saw the same thing – my shape. What I discovered was that although my shape was still the same, my SIZE was not! Talk about an eye opener! Another shock for this scale addict!

This is only the beginning of my new journey. I still have goals to meet, but that's the way I like it. It gives me something to work toward. I'll always have that next leg of my journey. I'm a work in progress and that motivates me! And when life throws me a curveball, I know that it won't derail me. I just work through it, and go back to where I was before.

What matters most is that I have officially broke free from the scale and am now ready to take part in the next challenge.

I have never felt more amazing, vibrant, healthy, energized and alive!

Gone are the negative thoughts and the jello-jiggler wiggle. I am a new me and proud of it!

My experience with Fit Yummy Mummy at this point is not so much about what I lost, but rather what I gained!

I gained an incredible amount of respect and knowledge about myself. I learned how strong I am both internally and externally. And most importantly, what I found during this transformation was something that I didn't even know I was looking for at the beginning......ME."

- Niki Baklund, Age 31, Mom of 8 year old son; Hutchinson, Minnesota – Fit Yummy Mummy since January 2011 and Proud Member of ClubFYM

Just like Niki, I too used to give the scale way too much power. Looking back I see that not only did this number dictate the mood of my day, it also lead me to engage in unhealthy habits that gave me the false sense that I was able to be in control of keeping this number as low as possible. This exhausting routine only resulted in damaging my metabolism and even worse, my self-esteem. Looking back I now see that I was a slave to the scale and I truly am more than just a number.

Now to help you get past this obsession with the scale, I'd like to ask you a question.

Ready?

"Would you like to weigh less or take up less space?"

Take a moment to really think about this one. You are all here to lose FAT, right? In order to make this happen there are fundamental fat loss factors that must be in place - eating supportively, effective strength training plan, intervals instead of long hours of cardio and of course, an attitude programmed for success.

The most unfortunate part of the fat loss process is that many women give up, quit and believe they are destined to be overweight, for they cannot get the scale to budge. This is a devastating path to take and can be very easily avoided when you simply understand what is happening, and know what to look for.

Why is the Scale an ineffective measure of success?

It CANNOT show you the change in your body composition - the loss of fat and the increase in lean muscle. As you gain some lean muscle and lose some fat, the numbers on the scale do not initially change....but magically, your clothes are no longer snug - what is happening?

First let me quickly clear up the Muscle vs. Fat Controversy

Pure fat is around 0.9g per cubic centimeter, while muscle is around 1.1g per cubic centimeter.

In other words....muscle is leaner and tighter than fat.

And yes, muscle is super-important to your body-shaping goals. Increasing your lean muscle:
1. Burns More Fat
2. Boosts your metabolism
3. Allows you to fit comfortably into your skinny jeans
4. Increases your Strength
5. Increases bone density
6. Makes you look lean, toned and defined

When fat is decreased on the body and slight muscle gains take place by following a full body-strength training program, it creates a more fit, lean, toned and attractive look.

It's past time to get off the scale. Why would anyone put all this effort into changing how to eat, how to workout and how to live each and every day for nothing in return? No one would. But we all crave and NEED some type of feedback. Crazy cool thing is - You already have it!

Throughout your weight loss efforts, have you at one time or another noticed....
• A melting away of inches
• A barrage of compliments - others are noticing a pleasant change not only in your appearance but in your overall attitude
• A tremendous amount of Energy
• The ability to DO more than you ever could before
• An amazing amount of Self Confidence

Now, another question for you.... Has a scale EVER given you the feedback I have just listed above?

No, and it never will. Stop beating yourself up and step OFF the scale.

Instead focus on what DOES measure and create momentum for successful results.

How?

Take circumference measurements, use your skinny jeans and take "before" pictures. Why? Because you can see them. As your fitness level improves, as your strength increases, as you drop a jean size, does it really matter what the scale says?

If you really think about it, a rational person would be totally willing to gain a few pounds in exchange for losing an inch in their soft and squishy spots. Get this...my body today – after 2 babies – is now 16 pounds heavier than when I was addicted to the scale and doing everything I could to control this number.

Just like so many other things that have changed in my life as I have found my passion and paved the way for Fit Yummy Mummy to reach moms around the world, so did this! My scale has been retired for a while and it has been one of the best things I've done. It is my hope that you too will put it up for a time and focus on the changes that truly matter to your long-term results.

At the end of the day, it's your life that can change the scale, not the other way around.

Change your perspective to something healthier – change your body forever!

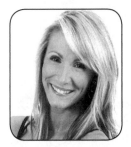

About Holly

Holly Rigsby is The Fit Yummy Mummy and Busy Mom Fat Loss Expert.

Holly is an ACE certified personal trainer, Kettlebell Athletics Certified and author of FitYummyMummy.com the 16 Week Fat Loss System designed Exclusively for Busy Moms, helping moms burn the baby fat with 15-minute workouts that can be performed at home. Holly launched this exciting fat loss plan for Moms in 2007 after going through her own personal post baby transformation.

Holly has since created a number of fat loss tools in an effort to simplify body-shaping results for moms, including the comprehensive Transformation Kit complete with follow- along workout DVDs, Intervals for Busy Moms with soundtracks and follow-along videos as well as a Fit Yummy Mummy Cookbook.

She is also the founder of ClubFYM.com ~ The Best Online Support Community for Moms. Moms meet online to get connected, feel supported and successfully transform their bodies by taking part in Transformation Challenges, personally interacting with Holly and receiving 2 new fat-burning workouts each month with follow-along videos.

Holly graduated from the University of Louisville with a Masters of Arts in Teaching. She has worked with over 11,000 Mom's to help them lose the stubborn baby fat and get and even better pre-baby body back. As a trainer, friend and coach, it is Holly's mission to educate, motivate and inspire women to take action and go after their dreams and goals.

For more information about Holly and the fat-loss programs and support she has to offer, plus grab a free "*Get Your Body Back Starter Pack*," visit her blog at: www.GetFitAndYummy.com or send an email to: Holly@FitYummyMummy.com

CHAPTER 12

Kaizen Fitness and the Hedgehog Concept: A Model for Long Term Fitness Planning

By Timothy J. Ward

"The fox knows many things, but the hedgehog knows one big thing."
~ The Greek Poet Archilochus

I was first introduced to the idea of hedgehog concepts when I read the book Good to Great by Jim Collins. It is a business book which, through empirical research, was able to detail what exactly it is that transforms a good company to a great one.

At the core of a great business is what Collins refers to as "the hedgehog concept," but before I can explain what that is and how it relates to The Fit Formula, I must first relate to you the story of the hedgehog and the fox.

The Hedgehog and the Fox

In 1953, an essay written by Isaiah Berlin was published that was titled The Hedgehog and the Fox. Despite the fact that the essay was originally written to analyze the author Leo Tolstoy and his works, the essay became what is considered by many scholars to be among the greatest ever written. This is not merely because his analysis of Tolstoy was so profound. What makes the essay famous is the way Berlin's analysis of a simple quote can be extrapolated to effectively mark the difference that divides human beings into two distinct categories.

Foxes are cunning, crafty creatures. They know a great deal of things, and they are often described as devious. However, for all that they know and for all the strategies they can come up with, when they try to hunt hedgehogs, they are powerless.

This is because the hedgehog simply knows one big thing.

Day-in and day-out the fox comes up with a new plan to make a meal of the hedgehog. He circles around the hedgehog's den just waiting for the perfect moment to pounce. When the hedgehog leaves his den to find food, the fox has his chance, and he leaps out hoping to surprise and kill the hedgehog using his new plan.

Of course the hedgehog, although in danger, is not afraid. He wonders if the fox will ever learn. The hedgehog rolls up into a ball and becomes a sphere of sharp spikes. The fox sees this and realizes he is beaten; if he moves in for the kill, he will simply get speared. So he retreats and returns the following day with a new plan. Yet for every new day and every new plan, the hedgehog remains unbeaten.

The problem with the fox is that it is his nature to see the world for all its complexities, and therefore, he will try everything he can think of to get what he wants. Despite wanting to hunt and kill the hedgehog, a fox can never become great at doing so.

The hedgehog, meanwhile, knows one big thing. It is self-aware, in a sense, because what it knows is simply what it is: a hedgehog. All the hedgehog needs to do is turn into a ball of spikes and remain a ball of spikes until the fox retreats, and it will prevail.

Collins took this concept and related it to the success of businesses. Those businesses that were able to identify their hedgehog concept, that one big concept that made them what they were and defined what they were good at, and then relentlessly pursue it were the ones who were able to make the leap from good to great. Those that continued on scattered and inconsistent, were the ones that either failed to make the jump or collapsed entirely.

Bruce Lee once said, "I fear not the man who has practiced 10,000 kicks once, but I fear the man who has practiced one kick 10,000 times."

It is my assertion to you that this same idea can be applied to the success of your fitness program.

My belief is that there are two kinds of "exercisers." There are those people, and you may know some of them, who bounce around from program to program and diet to diet, trying dozens upon dozens of different methods that are supposedly designed to get them to lose fat, pack on muscle, or whatever else people are after.

There are very few people who have never heard a friend or family member say, "I've tried absolutely everything, but I just can't _____." These are the foxes. The real truth of the matter is that most of these people have tried everything save one, and that one thing is what always seems to work.

The other "exercisers" are your hedgehogs, and they embrace, whether consciously or not, another philosophy entirely.

Kaizen Fitness

The Japanese call it kaizen, and the concept was first utilized success-fully in Japanese business practices. The philosophy has since been implemented in many other venues including healthcare, government, banking, and even fitness. The International Youth Conditioning Asso-ciation (IYCA) and the youth fitness franchise Athletic RevolutionTM integrate kaizen into both their foundational teachings and their long-term athletic development practices.

Kaizen is simply translated to mean "improvement" or "change for the better." The kaizen philosophy is designed to eliminate waste, because those who apply it practically will actively pursue improvement in all aspects of their lives.

Despite the linguistic bridge I may have just built, kaizen is not a new concept in fitness by any means. Fitness professionals and exercise en-thusiasts who have not lost sight of the big picture in favor of the latest industry fads and trends, simply call it progression.

It can go by other, fancier names as well, such as the overload principle, and it can be explained by the SAID principle (specific adaptation to imposed demands).

In my first book, The Theory of Fat Loss, I defined a training paradigm which I called The Theory of Absolute Intensity. It states, "The greater the absolute intensity one can achieve with training, the greater the fat loss result will be." Training until you are tired, as a means to an end, simply does not work unless it is accompanied by objectively measurable improvements in work capacity over time.

Looking back on it now, I see that I was merely shedding a different light on the progression concept. So, whatever you want to call it, however you want to explain it, and whichever way you wish to utilize it, ... is fine with me.

However, for those who value simplicity in its truest sense, simply take to heart the word kaizen and apply it to everything you do.

The Three Circles of Kaizen Fitness

I sometimes upset certain people when they ask me what I think of a certain exercise program or when they ask me what program is the best for _____. A lot of people seem to be convinced that there are these magical fitness formulas or brand new cutting edge concepts that only brilliant, divinely inspired, and larger than life figures can come up with that they have to buy for hundreds of dollars and follow along with for 90 days, or some other nonsense, or they won't get results.

The truth is that many different exercise programs and diets will help you reach your goals. Short of people telling flat-out lies, how else would so many different fitness programs be able to produce so many testimonials and successful transformation pictures? In fact, you could probably take any number of ideas or programs from any one of the esteemed authors of The Fit Formula and make them work, and I hope you choose to do so because there is a wealth of information inside this book from well-respected professionals in the industry.

The point is that the common denominator of fitness success does not lie within any one method or program. A program, no matter who created it, is not the primary factor which makes the difference between a person reaching fitness goals or failing. What I have come to understand is that there are three key dimensions to success or failure in fitness, and people who achieve success are able to translate (whether consciously or not) their understanding of the many potential aspects of these dimensions into a simple, profound paradigm that guides all their efforts. That paradigm is kaizen, our progression principle, the fitness hedgehog concept.

More precisely, kaizen fitness is a simple paradigm that relates all the complexities among the intersections of the following three circles:

1. Your mindset. Do you believe you have what it takes to be successful? Are there mental roadblocks preventing you from taking action towards the goal you have laid out for yourself? Almost all successful people eventually reach a point where they firmly believe in and enjoy what they are doing.

2. Your nutrition. Does your nutrition plan align with your exercise program and match your goal? Are you consistent with your nutrition, or are you standing in the way of your own success? The most successful fitness stories come from those who discovered a way to avoid being "dieters" and who have instead embraced healthy nutrition habits and lifestyles.

3. Your exercise program. Do you look forward to your training days? Is your exercise program something that you can actually improve within over time, or will you just be doing the same thing day in and day out, getting tired but not making objective progress? Successful people almost always enjoy what they do and have a way to show objectively measurable progress within their exercise programs, no matter what that program is, over time.

If the kaizen fitness principle is applied wholeheartedly to all three circles and their intersections, the fitness goal will be achieved. The key to building a lasting success does not lie in the application of kaizen to merely one or two of them, but applying it to all three circles.

If you have a great mindset and believe that you will achieve success and follow a fantastic program where you continually improve at what you are doing, but don't work to improve your diet, you may get results for a little while, but you will not build lasting success.

Similarly, if you work hard to improve your diet and develop all the right habits while consistently reaching personal milestones in the gym but are miserable, dread every day, hate everything that you do, and don't believe in what you are doing, you will eventually fall apart and will either fail to reach your goal or not be able to sustain whatever it is that you do end up achieving. However, if you improve a negative attitude little by little every day, surround yourself with a great social support structure to keep you motivated, and find a way to look forward to what you do while embracing what you are trying to accomplish, then you will be able to achieve a lasting success that is truly worth admiration.

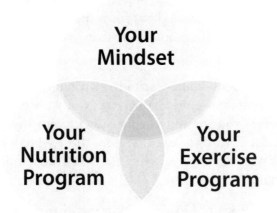

The Three Circles of Kaizen Fitness
Change for the better: Progression in all three circles day by day
will enable you to reach your goals

Long Term Fitness Practical Planning

Now that you understand the framework that needs to be in place, how do you actually go about taking action, and how do you know what you'll need to do? While different people may have other ideas, I think it is valuable to start by thinking about "the finished product." That is, who is the ideal you? It is not important whether you think this ideal will change or not, as it most assuredly will once you reach your goal. It is simply just important that you have established some lofty goal to work towards.

Now, if you have not already transformed into the ideal person you are

KAIZEN FITNESS AND THE HEDGEHOG CONCEPT: A MODEL FOR LONG TERM FITNESS PLANNING

picturing, then rather than just thinking about this while you read, I implore you to grab a pen and paper or computer of some sort and write out plainly and precisely the answer to that question. Once you are done, start breaking that person down by answering the following questions about the three circles. Of course, if you need help filling in some details, I encourage you to seek the advice of a qualified fitness professional or look for some of the answers within this book.

1. What does this person's exercise program look like? How often does this person train, for how long, and how hard? What movements is he or she performing? How strong, fast, or talented is this person in these movements?

2. How does the 'ideal you' eat? How often does he or she eat? What types of foods is this person eating, and which foods is this person avoiding?

3. What types of people surround this ideal person? Is this person happy? Does he or she look forward to the challenges of each day? Does this person have self-confidence?

Finally, compare these answers to the current you. This comparison will provide you with a blueprint showing where you are now and where you need to make progress to become the 'ideal you.' Every day, if you apply the kaizen principle within each of the three circles, then over time, you will achieve whatever fitness success you are after.

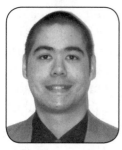

About Timothy

Timothy Ward graduated from the University of Notre Dame in 2009 at the age of 20 and is now a fitness business consultant with Fitness Consulting Group. Tim is the author of the 2010 book The Theory of Fat Loss: A New Paradigm for Exercise and served as editor for Pat Rigsby's The Little Black Book of Fitness Business Success. He has also done editing work on certifications for the International Youth Conditioning Association and Resistance Band Training.

In addition, he serves as the Vice President of Operations for two franchised fitness businesses, Fitness RevolutionTM, the world's fastest growing personal training franchise, and Athletic RevolutionTM, the only personal training franchise dedicated exclusively to the needs of young athletes aged 6-18, and is in charge of creating, managing, and disseminating the content of their subsequent franchise operations manuals.

For more information on Timothy Ward, visit his website at http://thetheoryoffatloss.com or add him to your circles on Google+ by visiting: http://gplus.to/timward

CHAPTER 13

The First Step to Fitness Success

By Pat Rigsby

A journey of a thousand miles begins with a single step.
~ Lao-tzu

Do you have a fitness goal that you want to pursue? Are you finding it difficult to take that first step toward making this goal a reality? What's holding you back? What has stopped you from taking those first steps to fitness or fat loss success? Here are a few things that have affected me at one time or another in the past:

Feeling Overwhelmed. Read the Lao Tzu quote again. 'A journey of a thousand miles begins with a single step.' No matter how large or how small the endeavor, you still have to begin with a single action. You don't have to have it all figured out. Simply take the first step.

Fear of (Fill in the blank.) It could be any number of things. Failure. Humiliation. Loss. Odds are the fear that you're experiencing is far worse than the actual reality – if whatever you're afraid of did happen. 99% of the time, the fear that's holding you back is not that big of a deal. The potential discomfort you'd experience is nothing compared to the elation you'd experience from actually achieving your goal.

Unwilling To Leave The Comfort Zone. This is just a nicer way of saying you're being too lazy to reach your goals. You must accept that achieving anything of significance requires work and dedication. So log out of

Facebook, quit texting, and hop off the couch and make your dreams happen.

Comparing Ourselves With Others. Your objectives should simply be tied to reaching your own potential. Don't worry about other people and what they've done unless it fuels you to work harder and do more. Otherwise focus on being the best version of you.

Thinking Things Had To Be Perfect. Waiting until the situation is perfect is a direct route to inaction because the situation will never be perfect. No matter how well prepared you are, there will always be something unexpected that pops up, so don't let the need for perfection stand in your way.

Doing More Research. This is just another way of saying "you're too lazy to do the real work." As I just mentioned, things don't have to be perfect to get started, so the need for endless research before taking action is completely unfounded.

Not Feeling 'Worthy' Enough. Not believing that you had enough education, knowledge, skill or experience can stop you before you get started, but the truth is that you can't get experience without 'doing' and you can't develop your skill without practice. Most every 'expert' I know felt this way at one point or another and still proceeded to take action. So should you.

If you're like me, the seven things that I listed above have at one time or another stood between inaction and action. But they're all just small obstacles designed to separate 'the haves' from 'the have-nots'… the successful from the average. The real bottom line is this: no matter what your goal, the best time to start is now.

I learned this back when I became a college baseball coach at the ripe old age of 23. At that point I was the youngest collegiate head coach in the country and felt a version of all seven things I listed previously:

- Becoming a head coach was completely overwhelming for someone who'd just graduated college a few months before. Being responsible for over 30 young men and a collegiate athletic program was far more responsibility than I ever had before.

- I was afraid of failure and humiliation. The program had never had a winning season prior to my taking over, in spite of being led by two well-known and previously successful coaches, so the odds were stacked against me, and I was worried about doing so poorly that I'd be fired and ruin any chance of getting another job in coaching.

- It's easy to say, "I'd like to be a college coach," but actually stepping up and applying and potentially being rejected was something that I struggled with.

- I looked at all the coaches of the programs I'd be coaching against, and it was obvious that they were far more experienced, more knowledgeable and had superior resources. I also took notice of the two previous coaches who held the position that I was applying for and recognized that by most any standard, they were far superior to me as a coach.

- I knew that the circumstances I was potentially entering were not ideal. A program with poor resources, a limited budget and no track record of success wasn't exactly the ideal launching pad for a successful career.

- Most 23-year olds that were interested in being a baseball coach were taking positions as Assistant Coaches for High School JV Teams, not going after Collegiate Head Coaching jobs. Why should I be any different?

But ultimately I accepted the premise above: ***the best time to start is now!***

And I learned as I went. When I started coaching, I didn't know how to run a practice, how to motivate players or how to recruit effectively. But I accepted the challenge and started the job anyway. The first few months were really tough. After my first season, I still hadn't 'found myself' as a coach. We had a winning season (barely), the first in school history in my first year, but it was more of a 'throwing stuff against the wall to see what sticks' approach than actually figuring things out.

Thankfully, the experience taught me a lot. The next year the team did better. ...By the third season, we were nationally ranked, and in the fifth season we finished 5th at the World Series.

And none of this would have happened unless I took the first step – in spite of my insecurities.

And what I learned through that experience has benefited me time and time again.

No matter what your goal, success is a process and it requires overcoming "limiting" beliefs and taking action.

Maybe your goal is to lose 30 pounds of unwanted weight. …Perhaps it's to fit back into your 'skinny jeans' again this fall or to run a 10K race in the Spring. Maybe your goals are loftier. You might want to run a marathon or win a 5K. Maybe you want to compete in a powerlifting meeting or a figure competition. You might even want to follow your passion and move into a career as a fitness professional, and even have your own byline in a popular magazine.

It really doesn't matter whether you want to lose 10 pounds or 100, or walk your first 5K or win your next half-marathon. Actually, I'd encourage you to 'dream big' and set lofty goals for yourself. That's part of what makes life worth living. But you must understand, the key isn't so much what the goal is, but how you act on it.

Once you've set your goal, big or small, you will do much, much, better if you spend more time thinking about your 'first steps' than only the big picture dreams and goals that you've laid out.

Just recently, while doing a coaching session with a client of mine, I suggested that in addition to the big dreams he had set out for himself, I wondered if he might also benefit from having some realistic goals for the short term. I then proceeded to suggest a few.

While I don't know your particular 'big goals,' here are a few examples of first step goals that will help you generate momentum and start making real progress toward where you want to get to:

- If you want to run a 10K but are new to running, consider beginning with a light jog to the end of the street followed by 30 minutes of brisk walking.

- If you want to lose 50 pounds, start with doing 30 minutes of exercise each day.

- If you want to overhaul your diet, start by making one change like committing to eating a supportive breakfast every day.

- If you want to do a triathlon but are just starting out, commit to biking, swimming and running each twice per week.

To someone who has been exercising for quite some time, like an advanced runner or a competitive triathlete, these kinds of goals might seem rather small and insignificant – but for a newbie they'd be a good start. For someone who is just starting but is not deconditioned, these smaller goals might also seem a little insignificant also, however, I'd argue that to get to your 'big dreams' there are a lot of steps in-between.

And many of those steps might not be as exciting or as fun to think about as the big endpoint you've identified as your ideal destination. But often it's important to focus on the very next steps that you need to take, in order to move towards your goals. This is how you generate momentum. …By putting one foot in front of the other. …By getting up to workout in the morning when you don't feel like it. …By eating a healthy breakfast when doughnuts sound far better.

Success isn't a big leap. It's the combination of hundreds or even thousands of little steps in succession. Unfortunately, most people don't recognize that, so they look for the magic bullet, …the quick fix. And while this isn't good news if you're looking for immediate gratification, it's great news if you're willing to start stepping. And that's because you understand that the magic is in the process, and the process begins with that first step.

And don't think that you're stuck taking what you may feel are baby steps for long. Once you've achieved these first small goals, start to increase them. You might want to go from jogging down the street to running around the block, …then for a mile without stopping, …then another. Before you know it, you've put a series of steps together and you're well on your way to achieving your big goal.

But before you can run, you need to walk.

So, to quote Dr. Denis Waitley ~ *"There never was a winner who was not first a beginner."*

The most important thing you can do to make your goals a reality is to make that first step!

About Pat

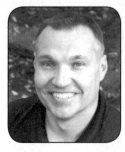

Pat Rigsby is an author, consultant and fitness entrepreneur as well as the Co-Owner of over a dozen businesses within the fitness industry. His company, the Fitness Consulting Group, is the leading business development organization in the fitness industry. The Fitness Consulting Group provides resources, coaching programs and consulting, to give you everything you need to start or grow your personal training or fitness-related business.

In addition to his business coaching and consulting work, Pat is also the Co-Owner of two of the leading youth fitness and sports performance companies in the world, Athletic Revolution and the International Youth Conditioning Association.

Athletic Revolution, the fastest-growing youth fitness and sports performance franchise in the world, was founded due to the need to provide fitness professionals, who sought to serve the Youth Fitness & Sports Performance market, with a systematic approach to developing a successful business – one that could provide them with the type of career they are seeking, while allowing them to have a profound impact in their community, serving the youth market. You can learn more about the Athletic Revolution Opportunity by going to: www.MyAthleticRevolution.com.

The International Youth Conditioning Association is the premier international authority with respect to athletic development and youth-participant-based conditioning. An organization that validates research and provides appropriate examples of practical application for working with young athletes and youth participants at large, the IYCA's goal is to enhance the knowledge of youth sports/ fitness professionals and volunteers throughout the world, via intensive educational opportunities as well as continuing education requirements. You can learn more about the International Youth Conditioning Association by going to: www.IYCA.org.

Pat also hosts a number of conferences, webinars and writes a blog and newsletter that reach over 65,000 fitness professionals on the topics of fitness-business development, fitness-marketing, and other business topics. He has been seen on NBC, ABC, CBS and in the pages of industry publications like Personal Fitness Professional, Club Industry and Club Business International. You can learn more about Pat's coaching programs and products, or download his collection of free business-building gifts by going to: www.FitBusinessInsider.com.

CHAPTER 14

The Power of Intention

By Dean Coulson

My Story

A long time ago when I was a lot younger, my Mam was really ill. I don't have many memories of it. I suspect I blocked it out because I was at a young age. No one likes to see a loved one suffer.

These days, my Mam is a lot better than she was back then, but still doesn't have the best quality of life (in my eyes), with vices in abundance and medication to "see her through." Her life experiences years ago have dictated her beliefs to this present day, even to the point that in recent years I have tried to help her, but she continues to choose not to accept the help I have offered.

Even though I wasn't really into sports too much at school, it was at this time that my Mam was ill. Looking back, it was the same time I started to take an interest in martial arts. I threw myself into it, pushing myself through each grading and trying to excel at everything. Then I also started to realise that there was more to martial arts than punching and kicking, so I explored more and more into fitness, and educating myself, trying everything out and finding my own way.

A few years ago, I was talking to some friends and I was asked why I was so driven when I trained. However, I could not answer the question, I did not know the answer! The reference was made about how I would (and still do) push myself and push myself to work and train harder. All I knew was that if I could do something in one session, I could better it in another. This applied to more than just training however, I also wanted to know as much about being healthy as I could, so I read dozens of nutrition books. The more I read, the more informed I was to make healthier choices.

Getting back to the question that my friends asked me, as I said I had literally no answer to it, it stopped me in my tracks and made me analyze and back-track, and it made me think about why I pushed myself so hard. I had to find the answer.

Now you may be wondering what this has to do with intention? Well I worked out why I was so driven. I didn't want to be like my Mam. I didn't want to suffer, I didn't want her to suffer anymore. I wanted to be as fit and healthy as I could be and so set about that goal in earnest. I then realized that my being healthy wasn't enough, I had to help others to be healthy, even if they didn't know it yet.

I had my intention. My desire and passion was so strong that I made my goal happen. Let me say this right now, if your intention is massive, so big that it consumes your every thought and you have passion and desire to follow it through, then the universe will conspire to help you.

Never has that been truer than over the last few years. Help has appeared when I have asked for it, from the most unlikely of sources. The reason for that is Intention.

Your Intention

So let me ask you this. How often have you wanted to do something, but something always got or gets in the way? It happens to many people about a great many things – bigger house, bigger car, more money, lose weight, get fit or own the gym of your dreams. The thing is, these things are end products, they are GOALS if you will – which are really rewards. They come about when you move 'hell and high water' to achieve something else that allows you to get your reward and realize your goal.

What about wishing you could do something, be something, go somewhere. Do you want to open a gym? But there is a raft of "problems" to overcome that you just cannot see any way around. Do you want to be mentored by the best in the world, but think you cannot even leave the town you are in?

Everyone has desires and dreams, but if they are not coupled with a solid intention, it actually does the opposite of what you want it to do. It can even push your desire away from you. In our ignorance, life protects us and if we haven't built up the mental strength to handle what we want, life won't send us things that we are not strong enough to handle.

Anybody can achieve anything they want, but many lack the very thing that is standing in their way between their dreams and their desires.... Faith and Belief!

Faith and Belief are what stand in between you and living your dreams, unless you have the belief to do something and the faith to carry it through, then you will find a lot of obstacles in your path.

If you fully intend something to happen but it doesn't, it is usually because something bigger and better is waiting for you around the corner. At the time though, our consciousness isn't big enough to know. You need to make it bigger, expand your consciousness so that you can see the bigger picture so you are on the same frequency, and then things will become clear.

"Our dreams are only an intention away."

Here's the thing however, intention is a strange beast. Just because you intend to have something, the desire to carry it out, the faith and belief that whatever you intend to have comes to fruition, ask yourself this, can you actually handle it? You may question what I mean, I hear you say of course I can, but what I mean is that anybody wants to have their dreams realized, but have you really thought about the consequences of them?

For example, let's say you want the best gym in your town and you get it, have you really thought about everything else? ...the running costs? ...the equipment costs? ...staffing costs? ...getting the clients in? ... marketing? ...sales?

This is when your intention is tested, a lot of people will take a look at this road map and decide it is too much to overcome and may even think that it is impossible to achieve. However, you must remember, it isn't reaching your destination that allows you to think bigger. You need to go through the journey to handle it, to grow into that mentality, to expand your consciousness to allow yourself to be able to. If your journey is littered along the way with pitfalls and problems, then as long as you overcome them, then you will become strong enough to handle your dreams when you get there.

Put it this way, if someone handed you the gym of your dreams tomorrow, would you take it on knowing what you have just read?

Remember, it is not the hurdles or pitfalls that prevent us from reaching our goal, it is the fact that we fail to overcome them that keeps us where we are.

Everyone has the power to succeed; VICTORY is built into every living person!

The first thing that intention will trigger is how to get your dreams realized. Obstacles are there for a reason, they are there to highlight that you are not yet ready to handle your dreams, they are there as tests to see if your dream is really what you want. It may be that the cost is too high, or that certain obstacles that you come across let you know that the cost is too high, that the dream you thought you wanted to fulfil wasn't what you wanted after all.

For example, I have seen people so consumed by a dream and goal that everything else suffers, relationships break down and you find yourself questioning whether what you are doing is really worth the result. I have been there myself, it is easy to be consumed by what you want, just make sure it isn't to the detriment of everything else. Once you decide to follow this path, everything around you changes and affects everyone around you. You better make 'damn sure' that everyone dear to you is along for the ride, because the cost can be very high. What I am saying is this, it is great to have dreams, to go for your goals, believe that you can achieve them and have the intention to do so, but remember there always has to be a balance. Listen to your body, keep things in perspective, do not push and push and push until you breakdown. There is a lot of truth in work, rest and play, make sure you cover them all. Work hard, know when to back off and when to take yourself away from it all.

Don't be discouraged by obstacles though, they are there to challenge you to see if your intention is strong enough. The universe rarely allows us to put more weight on a barbell when we can lift, and it is the same with dreams.

In reality, you want the road you are travelling littered with obstacles, because it means it is a road less travelled. Keep away from the well-trodden roads because it means many before you have already been down that road.

You Gotta Ask!

How often do you think about luck, getting a bit of good luck, wanting some good luck, being lucky, thinking you are unlucky. The thing is, in my experience, you should just forget it. In this life you make your own luck. It is amazing how many things just fall into place when you least expect it, but when you need it most. …the people that can and will appear just when you need them most. A book, or even a chapter in a book that just opens up at exactly the right page to tell you what you need to hear at exactly the right moment.

It has happened to me many times in the last few years, in fact it happened to me last week, picking up one of my many books on my reading pile. I happened to open a book on a random page and the answer was there before me, no word of a lie. I manifested the answer! Once you realize that you can have what you want if you want it badly enough, or should you say if your intention is strong enough, then the universe will show you the way.

Remember, when you want to know something, just ask. If you are stuck, then ask. If you have a problem to overcome, ask. I am not a religious person. However, as the bible quotes "Ask and you shall receive, seek and you will find, knock and it shall be opened." So you know what to do, ask! Make sure you ask the right question, but be very clear on what you want; make sure every detail is clear, because you usually get what you ask for.

Remember, don't wait for things to come to you because they won't – you have to get out there and find them. Whatever you want, go and get it, but go with the belief that if you are happy with what it brings, and the cost to you (the sacrifices you may have to make, the time it may take you), you will find it as long as your desire is strong, you have the passion to pursue it, the belief that you can achieve it, and the intention to get there.

So remember, INTENTION is the key to holding everything together to achieve your desires, but be aware of the cost and accept it.

The Success Formula

1. Have the desire to follow your dreams, the faith and belief that you can achieve it, and the strong intention to carry them through to fruition.

2. It is all very well having a strong intention, but what is intention without the goals to achieve? Always be very clear on your goals and remind yourself of them daily.

3. There are times when the road gets difficult. Keep your inspiration alive by surrounding yourself by like-minded successful people and read books by inspirational people.

4. Remember that what you are doing has to be congruent with you and your vision. Don't deviate from your goals. Happiness is essential!

5. Keep things in balance. Know yourself and your body, be aware of how you feel and make sure you are healthy. You may need a break, whether that is an hour, a day or a week; take it or you will regret it if you don't.

6. Don't procrastinate, don't let fear get in the way. Fear is just an emotion, it is only real if you make it real. Always ask yourself whether what you are doing will harm you. What is the worst that can happen by doing what you are doing? As Susan Jeffers says, "Feel the fear and do it anyway," or as one of my mentors always says, "There is no growth in comfort. Marinate in fear, get used to being uncomfortable as a way of life."

7. The time to act is now. Do not get caught up in excuses why you cannot do what you want. You can do anything you want, it is you that are placing the shackles on yourself, get rid of them! Remember, the buck stops with you. Do not blame anyone else, accept responsibility for your own actions. When you blame something else you are giving that thing power over you, why do that? Change your perception and you can change anything!

The time to act is now, so Act!

About Dean

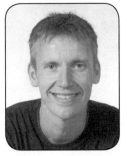

Dean Coulson is a fat loss expert and Health Coach in North East England. He is the owner of Assert Health and Fitness, offering one-to-one, semi-private training, group training, fitness camps and rehabilitation, helping hundreds of clients attain their fat loss and fitness goals.

He is a regular article contributor on various strength and conditioning websites, and regularly hosts discussions on various social media platforms for other fitness professionals and fitness enthusiasts around the world. He also regularly mentors other trainers in the UK and across the world in nutrition and training advice.

His blog: www.allroundathlete.com is viewed by thousands of people worldwide and contains all manner of information to help people achieve their own fitness goals.

He has been involved in the martial arts for 25 years, studied several martial arts to black belt level, and is a certified self-protection instructor, studying under the world renowned Geoff Thompson's real combat system through the British Combat Association.

His ambition is to run a facility which rivals the best in the world, serve as many people as possible, and educate them to a fitter, healthier lifestyle.

Find out more by visiting:
www.assert-fitness.co.uk
www.assert-selfprotection.co.uk
www.allroundathlete.com

CHAPTER 15

Your Personal Trainer Isn't So S.M.A.R.T.

By Mike Bach

Have you ever been in a position when you're right at the start of your "campaign" to get in shape, lose weight or compete at your best that you are bursting at the seams to get going, and that nothing will stop you – this time?

You might have one or several of methods in place to make sure that this happens – a goal, a gym membership, a new pair of running shoes, a personal trainer, a weight loss club membership or a stack of brand new off-the-shelf celebrity "tone-up" DVD's?

Whatever your preparation, it seems like everything you could ever need is in place to guarantee your continued progress to your dreams and desires. Doesn't it therefore make you wonder why your on-going actions do not speak as loudly as the desires you once started with?

You don't feel as attached to the goals that you once had, and struggle with the motivation to carry out the day-to-day processes that would automatically qualify you for results! Your thoughts and feelings are not as focused towards the idea that you once had about how your were going to look and feel, resulting in telling yourself lies like "I'll start Monday," or "Now's not the right time with everything else I've got going on," or "What I'm doing will work just as well," or "It's actually not that important to me!"

Sounds familiar, doesn't it? ...and that's because I've seen people and heard conversations like this from people that experience the merry-go-round of highs and lows – and inevitably lose their game. And I can tell you that it's a lot to do with the strategies of personal development that have been used over time; strategies that miss out one key simple but very influential ingredient.

Background

I've not always been the fitness coach that you now see in front of you in this book, and my background has largely been academic and then corporate up until 5 years ago. Always being a sports and fitness nut (my head was in these text books more than my management science course reading list), it was obvious that I was then going to sit down behind a desk for the next 10 years at university blue chips, right?

Okay, not entirely obvious, but that is exactly what I did do, and throughout that time I learnt a lot about goals, targets, deliverables, objectives and so on. The corporate organisation was crazy about wanting to teach you about how to set and achieve your deliverables as they were called in business, using what I now call the "Not So S.M.A.R.T. Method" when it comes to setting out and realizing your health and fitness goals.

If you don't already know, this is what a S.M.A.R.T. goal is.

S – The Specifics of the goal such as the main question of "What Do I Want To Achieve" but might also set other specifics such as what is the purpose and benefits of achieving the goal.

M – How to Measure the goal? How will you know when it is going to be achieved, what are the milestones, the dates?

A – Is the goal Attainable? The suggestion in this process is that while the goal should stretch the team/person to achieve them, they are not extreme and therefore meaningless.

R – Is the goal Relevant or Realistic? Are you willing and able to work towards it?

T – And finally, Timely. When will the goal be achieved by?

Through college, university, HR development workshops and project management meetings, I had S.M.A.R.T. goals drummed into me! They just loved the things! So when I made the leap of action towards my passion and ultimately my purpose within the health and fitness profession, one of the first things I got lectured on was the use of these S.M.A.R.T. methods to coach my clients, and in doing so, keep them on the track towards progress and the realization of their goals.

The problem I had now though was a simple one.

All this time I'd been using this method or a similar process, it was being done…

- In a corporate environment on business projects – improving sales, delivering new systems and so forth
- To improve and evaluate personal performance of individuals in a corporate environment

Overall, it was performed in a very logical and methodical way because it was all about the company. The company drove the goal whether it was the project or the person.

In a personal fitness environment I soon discovered that the same method was not working well enough. Where two people were highly motivated to the "getting started" process, why would one succeed and the other one fail? Was it as simple as willpower and determination, or was it more down to the goal development strategies used – or not used?

The process didn't work because people become unattached to goals whether they want to achieve them or not when it is about improving themselves, because the goal does not take into consideration the INDIVIDUAL!

S.M.A.R.T. goals are all about the goal, and what I have to do is to relate that goal as strongly as possible to the person, by considering WHY the goal is important. Not having this link is what pretty much always results in a failure of sorts, as well as the lack of motivation to follow through.

It wasn't the change in diet being too hard. It wasn't a lack of time. It wasn't a lack of knowledge of what to do. It wasn't having the drive that comes from the emotions of 'what makes you tick' to find the right solution and use it on a consistent basis. To some degree the goal was becoming irrelevant, because the person was not considered as part of the building process and their emotions in particular.

Lets get this right! We all have emotions – it is not something to be embarrassed about if you are a 6' 5", 18 stone rugby player or a stay-at-home mum. We all do things to make us feel better about ourselves. The number one rule of life is that we are looking for fulfilment.

The skinny guy wants to build up his biceps so he looks good, attracts girls and by doing that he feels good. The athlete wants to win for personal achievement and recognition, and that makes him/her feel good. And any one of you that wants to lose 10, 20, 50, 100lbs to look good and attractive also wants those feelings as well.

So if we've got this demand for brilliant feelings, would it not make sense to have a plan and a set of strategies that use the power of these emotions and the individual to achieve so much more? Of course it would!

That's why I believed from the outset there was a better method to pursue personal success rather than being so logical about it. I estimate that at least 80% of what we achieve is by understanding our psychology, and the rest is made up of the mechanics of what we do.

Whether you know you're using a S.M.A.R.T. approach or just winging it, the same problem exists! There is no use for the real reasons and real energy that is in you to provide the biggest impact on your health and fitness desires. Just the fact that most people get angry and frustrated when they fail shows that there are bigger emotions involved.

I've come across lots of tools and strategies; such as from Tony Robbins outside the fitness industry and Dax Moy within it. In fact, it is on one of my good friends, Dax's acronyms, that I base a lot of my other principles and strategies around goal achievement now.

The Q.U.E.S.T. approach is an altogether smarter approach to goal achievement, which is why I confess to not being that S.M.A.R.T. at all!

Step 1 – "Q"ualify what it is that you REALLY, REALLY want?

From the offset forget about what is realistic! Who decides what is realistic? We are dealing with you as a person and not a corporate entity, right? Therefore we are dealing with emotions and excitement builds up that emotion, right?

Lets say you're 50lbs overweight. The protective instinct might be to say I'd be happy losing a stone. What's exciting about that? Will you really care about it enough that you'll follow through consistently? Probably not, and you'll still be angry and frustrated and not figure out why?

While I'm sure you'd be happy with that where's the excitement in comparison to wanting to lose 50 lbs and the changes that would happen to your health and you as a person, as a result? Don't be put off by the size of the task. Have the right reasons for doing something and the size does not matter.

And lets just say you don't reach your target and only get 80% of the way. Based on 14 or 50 lbs, that's still an extra 30 lbs, even if you reached the modest target of a stone. I don't think I'd be unhappy with that sort of failure!

The other side of the coin here is that what you really, really want is outside of your personal health and fitness, but for now stick with staying in this field of interest and the next part of the process will work that one out for you.

Help define your Q's by having a go at what your VISION is - lets say for in 12 months time. Your goals are simply a collection put together that then detail your vision. This helps you come up with anything and everything until you come up with what you really want.

Based on your vision can you qualify what you want and start to think about WHY you want it – what's so important about achieving that? Ask yourself further questions like what will happen as a result of achieving the goal, or better yet, what will happen if you don't achieve it.

Such questions help determine the significance of what you're chasing, and whether you still qualify them as desirable! The principle of SMART goals has been accomplished in one step – lets move on to the real money steps now!

Step 2(a) –
"U"nderstand WHY you want to achieve this(these) goal(s)

Most people are closed doors when it comes sharing with others their emotions, and to be honest, probably with themselves as well. One thing you should understand 100% is the real TRUTH behind why you want to achieve your fat loss and performance goals.

Wanting to look good for your holiday and the likes are not bad places to start, but then ask yourself why is it important to look good on holiday. Be 100% honest and come clean with yourself. And keep asking yourself WHY, to find deeper reasons and therefore more significant ones that will align you with the goals you have just set out (or not – in which case re-Qualify)!

Do you remember the Quan in Jerry Maguire that Cuba Gooding Jr. used to show the difference between getting the big coin and getting the whole package? This is the same, and if you don't already know it, what you are looking for. When a member comes up to me and tells me their success story, not only have they achieved the big weight loss, but also achieved many other things that they set out to do. …Better relationships and confidence, happiness in general and specific events, reversal of previous health complications, look younger, more energy, career success, increased turnover of personal business and the list goes on.

A bit more than losing 50lbs! This is what I call the M.T.V. Effect (Massive Transformation Value), and can provide some real clues into why the goal is so important. What else will happen as a result?

No one really cares about losing 50 lbs – it's the output as a result that matters, and therefore what is the driving force into your desires and essentially your personal fulfilment.
• Ask yourself what a typical perfect day would look like?
• Would the New You be part and parcel of that?
• Would the New You affect that?

It's becoming a bit more than a goal now! What we're doing is getting the goal to fit YOU! One that you also CARE about!

Step 2(b) – "U"nderstand WHERE you are right now

Part 2 of understanding is identifying the problems as they are right now between getting to your goal and everything else.

• Attach more of you to the goal by understanding why you are not there right now?

• What's stopping you?

• What are your angers and frustrations?

- How does being where you are right now negatively affect all the goals and desires you have?

- How does being where you are at right now have an impact on everything else that is part of your M.T.V?

Step 3 – "E"ducate yourself

- What are the new commitments?

- What do I have to change in order to get to where I REALLY want to get?

- You might not have all the answers now, in which case the first education would be to find someone who does, but have a go at building as detailed a list as you can.

Again, evaluate the goal for YOU and vice versa!

- Ask yourself whether you are you willing to make these new commitments?

And what are you not willing to do is just as important.

Part of this process is testing that the WHY's and WHERE's are big enough to ensure you are willing to commit to new ways. Part of the big issue with other methods is that they fall over because you stop being willing even though the pain of where you are at right now disappoints you. They key is that you're already invested in both the exciting goal and the MTV effect it will bring.

Could you really afford not to commit now knowing the real reasons as to why it's so important and what it will bring when it works for you?

Step 4 – "S"timulate

If you don't already have excitement (I have!) stimulate it more! The truth is, as time goes on, we can all forget about what road we are on if we do not continue to excite ourselves with the challenge ahead and the rewards it will bring.

We need to remind ourselves to create that emotion we had when first going through the steps above using strategies from the off. Visualise what it will look and feel like. Create a vision board!

Share with others – talk about what you are doing with others. Create excitement and accountability. Share with yourself – tell yourself out loud in the form of incantations. Movement and being audible bring what's on the inside to the outside, creating more energy. If you have more energy, you create more positive emotion and with that come consistent actions.

Undertake some research. One of the big exciting WHYS for one of my clients was to get into the fitness profession to define her purpose and how she could help more people. One of the first things she did was research how this would become possible – what courses to do, who provided the best fit and she started to go to conferences on the specific subject matter that interested her.

Create happiness! When anyone tries to change, it can be from a place that is currently unfulfilling, and when you're not fulfilled your energy drops and action taking does the same – that's why many people overeat – they think they need fuel when all the need is energy! Promote more energy and fulfilment by not just changing your psychology but your physiology, and get active as well as visualising. See the energy levels change and the attitude as well.

Step 5 – "T"est all the time

Do you still qualify for the goal and does the goal still qualify for you? More about qualifying if you're getting picky but worthy of testing, so that your sat nav is still pointed towards the right location. Evaluate whether it is still important!

I like the idea that we never reach our goals! Why? Because we should be evaluating them and then changing them when we are almost there as a new challenge excites us.

Where are you now in relation to where you want to be? Mark it out of 10 and you'll probably find that as soon as you close in on a 10 that it becomes a 6 or 7 again!

Testing is good to help change the goalposts when required to maintain the momentum. I never reach a 10 and I'm not dissatisfied about that!

Before that happens though, test by way of milestones and measure your progress towards the ideal you. And give yourself challenges that you can test yourself with along the way, whether it is a certain weight by the end of the year or completing 10 full push-ups. As long as it follows the same theme of building the relationship between you and the goal!

Building your goals in a way you feel fulfilled isn't about trying to maintain the same motivation throughout the journey that you had when you first picked up your running shoes and new track top; it's about making sure that you have the right strategies in place, so that you can maintain high levels of performance of action taking even when dips occur.

So don't be as dumb as going S.M.A.R.T. or any other process that fails to harness the energy and potential that is within you, and use what's unique about you to stay attached, keep the drive, and inspire you towards the bigger picture.

You don't need a better time to start or another diet plan or the latest 6-minute abs routine; you need to understand you!

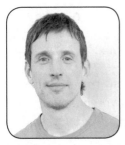

About Mike

Mike Bach is one of the UK's leading total body transformation experts encompassing physique, performance and internal health.

Operating out of South Manchester, Mike is the owner of Body Planner Fitness and a Nike-sponsored trainer. He is also the creator of the M.A.G.I.C. Principles and The Rich Body Rich Life Formula.

With these systems, Mike consults and coaches one-on-one, both locally and further afield, as well as owning a set of Fitness Camps across Manchester and Cheshire.

Working with a wide range of clients – from athletes and sports to general and from business owners/corporate clients to housewives, Mike is a firm believer that having great health is a must for getting the max out of your life and fulfilling your true potential professionally and personally. Mike does this time and time again by combining psychological, nutritional and physical principles.

Find out more about Mike, Body Planner Fitness and new developments at:
www.thebodyplanner.com
www.manchesterbootcamp.com
www.tenyearsyoungerplan.com

CHAPTER 16

The Fit Formula –

Because You're Worth It...

By Sam Feltham

Why do some people succeed and some people, in my eyes, temporarily fail in their health and fitness journey? Simply put, it's how you think, feel and act.

You see, I had a pretty tough time growing up as a kid. When I was 8 years old, my Father committed suicide leaving my Mother with 4 children, 2 girls and 2 boys, to bring up by herself. She is my true inspiration in life and why I have been able to become the man I am today.

But the icing on the cake was when I was 13 and was diagnosed with Hodgkin's disease, a mild form of cancer. The lymph node gland in the right side of my neck swelled up to the size of a small egg and my Mother took me to the doctor. He said that this happens to lots of teenage boys and that it was nothing to worry about, but of course my Mother knew better. We went back a second time and still he said it wasn't anything to worry about. The third time my Mother demanded that I was to have it biopsied and looked at.

All I can say is, thank god my Mother followed her intuition and kept to her guns, because if it weren't for her I wouldn't be here today to help you.

After my diagnosis, I was put on to a four and a half month course of chemotherapy. Thankfully, we caught it early enough and I was cleared after those four and a half months.

Another one of my greatest achievements to date is when I walked by myself from Lands End to John O'Groats, which is the length of Britain, a journey of 1000 miles. I ended up covering about 26 miles a day, a marathon, and completed the walk within 62 days. Now I'm not going to sugar coat it, it was tough and every step was difficult, but without the foundations of overcoming adversity from my youth, I'm not sure I could have completed that journey.

> *"The journey of 1000 miles begins with a single step"*
> ~ Lao Tzu

My inspirational Mother, my near death experience with cancer and the 1000 mile journey on foot have all given me a very good foundation for an achieving mindset, but most importantly, they've taught me one extremely valuable lesson, that my life is worth living!

Before I move on to truly helping you, I just wanted to say to you, I hope you realise that you are unique, that you are special and that you are worthy of having a long, healthy and abundant life.

As well as all the previously mentioned experiences, I have also been an international snowboard coach, coaching beginners to instructors in New Zealand, Switzerland, Austria, America and Canada. From all my years as a coach, whether it is in snowboarding or in health and fitness, I've come to one conclusion. 9 times out of 10 it's not that people lack the skill to achieve, it's just that they lack the self-belief that they can do it.

How do you increase self-belief?

When dealing with self-belief with my clients I like to talk about the 3 F's, forgiveness, fear and fact.

Firstly, you must forgive yourself. We are so quick to acknowledge our past mistakes and keep those in the forefront of our minds rather than our victories in life. I look at past mistakes like the drawer that you keep all the electrical wires in at home. You throw them in one by one, and after a while they all start to get tangled up. When the drawer is full and you can't put in any more wires, you get so angry with yourself that you didn't sort it out sooner and it becomes overwhelming to deal with.

If we had organized those wires from the beginning it would have made things a lot easier for sure. However, unfortunately for some of us, the tangled up wire drawer is overflowing from our past mistakes and would take years to untangle. Fortunately though, metaphorically speaking, most of the equipment that is used with all those tangled electrical wires has either broken or is out of date. So what I suggest is that you just throw it all out! Get rid of it and forget about it.

> *"Our past actions are who we were, our future actions are who we are going to be!"*

Whenever you get angry with yourself for a past mistake, I want you to repeat this simple phrase to yourself to make you forget about it. As well as using this phrase, I want you to start writing a victory journal.

Using a normal diary or notebook, I want you to record every single victory you have everyday. No matter how small or how big, write it down and congratulate yourself. It could be that you throw an apple core into a rubbish bin from the other side of a room, or it could be that you helped your company complete the biggest sale in history. If you get a positive feeling of accomplishment, record it and hold on to it.

Secondly, we must deal with fear. Fear holds us back from reaching our full potential by stopping us from taking action. It stops us taking chances, it stops us from doing what we truly want to do and it puts up barriers in the way of us succeeding in anything.

When I began as an international snowboard coach teaching beginner-snowboarders to turn for the first time, I found it fascinating. You see, when snowboarding on groomed snow, you have to put your weight on to the front foot to steer with the front of the board. There were some people who just went for it, throwing themselves down the mountain, and of course, they would fall over a few times but they'd pick themselves up and try again. After a few falls, they started to find their feet and balance points and started not to fall down at all, having a fantastic time on the snow. Then there were the people who were too afraid to put their weight on to their front foot, and sure enough they spent the whole day falling over, having a miserable time. After many years of experience, I managed to actually help coach people to overcome their fear of putting the weight on to their front foot and having a fantastic time instead of a miserable time, quicker and quicker.

The way I did it wasn't the traditional "JUST DO IT ALREADY," because I tried that at first and it never ever worked. I said to them "Everybody is afraid, including myself and the people turning already. But the difference is that they've managed to box their fear within their mind momentarily to enable themselves to put their weight forward and make the turn." This simple concept of 'boxing up' their fear seemed to work wonders.

That's what I want you to do with your fear of the road ahead in your health and fat loss journey. Box up that overwhelming fear of what and how much is to be done. Put it to one side in your mind and deal with the problem on a daily or weekly basis instead of thinking how long the road ahead is.

My third and final piece of the self-belief puzzle is to make it a fact. A fact that in your mind you have achieved your healthy lifestyle already. Many motivational speakers in the past have said if you want to achieve, you've got to get hungry and really want it; well unfortunately, I'm here to tell you that this is the incorrect way to go about achieving.

Let me ask you right now, would you rather want something or actually have something? I'm guessing you'd rather have it, right? To actually succeed in your fat loss and health journey you have to trick your mind into thinking it has it already. Wanting something actually promotes a thought pattern and feeling of not having it. I can prove this to you right now with a quick little exercise.

Say out loud or in your head if you're in a public place, "I want to be fit and healthy" ten times. Now say out loud or in your head if you're in a public place, "I am fit and healthy" ten times. Quite a difference, isn't there? Saying "I am" rather than "I want" is promoting a thought pattern and feeling of having, which is the final ingredient in self-belief. Having that unfaltering self-confidence that you have succeeded in your fat loss and health journey already will get you there a lot quicker than just wanting it.

In summary, to create more self-belief, you must forgive yourself for your past mistakes, realizing that your future actions are who you're going to be, not let fear get in the way by boxing it up and making it a fact that you have succeeded in your fat loss and health journey already.

Self-belief is a great starting block for you to realize that you are worth it, but sometimes faith in oneself isn't enough for long-term motivation. Over the years of my experience with coaching people around the world in snowboarding and with their health and fitness, I've noticed how people think and say things directly impacts on how they feel about something and ultimately how they are going to act upon it.

For instance, in February 2011 I decided to do a bit of a crazy stunt in London, one of many, I might add. I went for a 2-minute lie down on The Millennium Bridge in London, which is a pedestrian bridge over the River Thames between the Tate Modern Art Gallery and St. Paul's Cathedral. This might sound like I'm going mad here, but it was an exercise to push my own comfort zones. I was rather nervous before doing it, making up all sorts of negative fictitious scenarios in my head. "What happens if the police showed up and told me to move on, how embarrassing would that be?" These thoughts were making me feel embarrassed already, and I hadn't even done it yet!

However, I boxed up my fear, told myself it'd be ok and did it anyway. During the 2 minutes of lying down on a busy pedestrian bridge at lunch time in London I had many people look at me very strangely, one person even asking me if I was ok which was nice, but after the 2 minutes finished and I got up and walked away, you know what happened? Nothing! No one particularly cared, apart from that person who was checking if I was ok. So all of the embarrassing thoughts and feelings I had going through me before and during my crazy stunt were just a figment of my imagination, and there was nothing to worry about in the first place.

My thought of a negative fictitious scenario before my crazy stunt is called a thinking error. I was making up a false reality without trying it out first and then making a sound judgement from there.

What I want you to do when you start having a thinking error is to stop and ask yourself, "Is what I'm saying to myself a negative fictitious scenario?" For example, "Oh! This new diet and exercise program will never work." You are creating a negative fictitious scenario based on no evidence at all before you've even begun, and seriously dampening your potential to actually achieve your optimal health and fitness. A more constructive way to think about it is, "Although I'm not sure that this new diet and exercise program will work, I will give it my best and see if it actually works before I give up on it." Here, you are accepting that there is a possibility it may not work, but you are willing to give your best anyway to see if it works, which means you are more likely to actually take action and get results.

In conclusion, start off by believing in your self again, as you can do it. But this isn't enough. You need to start re-programming the way you think, which inherently affects the way you feel and act. You must embrace your negative thoughts then positively move forward. More importantly though, you must not create negative fictitious scenarios without trying it out first, because you are worth it!

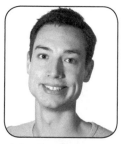

About Sam

Sam Feltham is the owner and head coach of Smash the Fat Fitness & Fat Loss Boot Camps, based in London, UK.

Sam has risen through the ranks of the health and fitness industry over a decade, starting out as a children's party co-ordinator in a sports centre, and working his way up to study at the European Institute of Fitness as a Master Personal Trainer, and becoming the owner of a successful fitness business in the UK.

Sam has come to be known as the 'Fat Loss Mindset Coach' within the health and fitness industry because of the many useful and productive workshops, seminars, articles, videos and products he has created.

To learn more about Sam, and to download his free book "7 Mindset Tricks of Highly Effective Fat Losers" – visit: www.FatLossMindsetCoach.com .

CHAPTER 17

The Fit Formula –
Your Journey of a Lifetime

By Nicky Sehgal

Success is a journey, not a destination. ~ Arthur Ashe

It's January 1st and you decide that this is it; this is the year you are going to begin your fitness lifestyle that you have always wanted. You've set your mind to exercise regularly, eat all the right foods and eliminate all the unhealthy lifestyle choices that has left you overweight, out of shape and feeling low on both energy and self-confidence.

It's the start of week one and your motivation is high, and you really think that this time you will get the results you crave. You get through the week; eat all the right food and religiously do a couple of workouts. Week two arrives and you manage to do the same, you feel good -- well done, you! Then something wonderful happens, you start to see some results, your clothes start to loosen up and you begin to feel amazing. Time goes on and before you know its week four and you still feel brilliant and say to your self, "Yes I can do this."

February comes along and life starts to get a bit busy and you begin to lose a little bit of your original enthusiasm and commitment that you had only a month ago. You begin to find that you are not working out as frequently as you were, and what's worse, you begin to eat on the run again.

Before you know it, it's March and your motivation levels are really starting to dwindle, its now becoming a chore to prepare all your healthy meals, and getting to the gym is becoming hard work. Soon you start to fall back into your old unhealthy habits. Your energy levels are dropping and you feel overweight and out of shape and begin to feel like you've failed, yet again.

If this sounds like you, don't worry. You're not alone and with the right tools you can prevent this from happening ever again. In the 12 years I have been a fitness professional, I have seen this scenario more times than not.

How many times have you started a new diet or fitness program only to find a couple of months into it you find yourself slowly drifting back to your old unhealthy habits? I bet it's quite a few, more importantly, why does this keep happening and what can you do so this never happens to you again?

I'm going to share some of my top strategies with you that I hope you can use to help develop a long-term fitness lifestyle. Whilst there is so much more than I could write in this chapter I am hoping that if you are willing to embrace my fundamental philosophies, based on my years of experience helping clients integrate fitness into their busy lifestyle and run with it, you will be on the right path.

Your Fit Formula Journey

You made a good choice by investing in this book, you have some of the world's best fitness trainers, nutritionists and coaches sharing their top strategies with you. All you now need to do is make a plan and get to work; yep, there is work involved. Nothing gets accomplished from just reading.

Before you start, I want you to understand that your fitness development is not going to happen in a straight line. In reality, there will be times when you are able to exercise more frequently and have better control of your diet. Equally there will most certainly be times in your life when you just can't exercise as much as you want and you have far less control of your diet. Things do happen in life and sometimes you will just need to 'take your foot off the gas' and just try to maintain your fitness. That's ok, but just don't stop and give up, even if you only manage to get in a single workout per week for a few weeks, just do it, and promise me that you won't stop altogether. Just keep moving forward, even if its at a snail's pace.

So what do you need to do to make fitness a permanent part of your lifestyle?

Here are some of my 'tried and tested' strategies that have helped me help others keep fitness as part of their lifestyle for a very long time and hopefully for a lot longer to come. As always, don't just read them, use them! Take massive daily action and you will reap the rewards of a healthier body and a happier you.

Your 7 Steps To A Fitness Lifestyle

1. Make This The Last Time You Start

It takes more energy for a shuttle to take off from its launch pad than it needs for the rest of its entire journey; the same is true for fitness. There is nothing harder in fitness than starting; it sucks, and it's hard. Ask any pro athlete what the most challenging part of their season is and they will always tell you its pre-season training camp. **Take a different mental approach to your fitness this time around, make this the last time you ever start a new weight loss or fitness program ever again. Because if you are always starting again, it means somewhere along the line you have given up, and we don't want that.**

Planned breaks are OK, it does not mean you have stopped, everyone needs a holiday from everything, even your fitness regime. You enjoy your break and let your body and mind recover and rejuvenate from your regime, but as soon as you can,get back and pick up where you left off

2. You Always Need To Work On Your Mind Set

The difference between people who manage to maintain a fitness lifestyle and those who don't normally comes down to their attitude and mindset; conditioning the mind is often an overlooked part of fitness by most people.

Here are a few ways you can help train your mind to become unbreakable.

- Dedicate some time to work on what you want out of your fitness regime and get it down on paper in the form of a goal. When you set your goals you instantly create a shift in your attitude to do the things you need to do to attain your goal. You must write down your goals and you must consistently review them and your progress towards them for them to have a positive conditioning effect on your mind.

- Surround yourself with others who already have adopted fitness as part of their lifestyle. We are heavily influenced by the people we spend most of our time with, we tend to pick up their habits whether positive or negative; so if you want to be fit surround yourself with people who stay in shape, it will help you keep on top of your fitness.

- Always think positive and recognise that no feat is beyond you – Always believe in yourself, there is no reason why you can't have what you want but you will only get it if you first believe in yourself.

- Read, listen and watch stuff which inspires you –– such as this book, fitness blogs, sports, inspiring stories, articles, etc., and as always, take action while your motivation is still hot.

Conditioning your mind so it's strong enough to overcome obstacles that will get in your way and keep you working on your fitness is something that you should not overlook, and you should consistently work on, no matter where you are on your journey.

3. Know What or Who Is Your Inspiration

There is nothing more powerful to keep your motivation levels high than having a continual source of inspiration. Being inspired and staying focused is one of my key strategies to help clients integrate fitness into their lifestyle long-term.

To find out what inspires you, ask yourself these questions:
• What has inspired you to get fit?
• Or who has inspired you to take up a fitness lifestyle?

It could be a number of things or people; the more things you have inspire you the better. If you know what inspires you it will provide all the motivation you need to keep you exercising consistently, keep your nutrition on track and keep you in good health.

Here's what inspires me.....

Just like you, I have my motivational ups and downs, but I know what inspires me to keep exercising and adopt healthy behaviours as an integrated part of my busy life. I love to see sporting victories, watch how dedicated athletes are, how they train, eat and live to reach their goal and ultimately their dream, their willingness to do what it takes to get them to the top, that's inspiring to me. If ever I'm lacking motivation, I may read quotes like this

Champions aren't made in gyms. Champions are made from something they have deep inside them: a desire, a dream, a vision. They have to have last-minute stamina, they have to be a little faster; they have to have the skill and the will. But the will must be stronger than the skill. - Muhammad Ali

That's powerful and its gets me to the gym all day long. Whatever your inspiration is, try to stay focused on this, integrate it into your lifestyle. Keep it where you can see it every day to remind yourself why you need to keep on top of your fitness.

4. Have someone to hold You Accountable

Having a trainer, coach or someone else hold you accountable is a great strategy to make sure you stick with your fitness lifestyle. All top professionals in any industry have coaches, teachers or managers to make sure they get the things that they need to get done to get them to the top. Its too easy to be lazy, its almost human nature to find an easier way to do things.

In fitness, this never works, only hard work will get you to the top, there are no short cuts.

If you don't want to hire a professional trainer, find someone who you are willing to discuss your goals with and ask them if you can report back to them on a weekly basis. These days you can do this online with a trainer for minimal cost, or join social groups for free. However you choose to do it, just do it, taking action is the key that will empower you to develop the fitness lifestyle you want.

5. Stay Consistent with your workouts: adopt the No Excuses Approach

This is almost a continuation from number 4, if you have some type of accountability you are likely to be more consistent and nothing will get you better results than staying consistent with your workouts and healthy lifestyle behaviours.

Here are my top five strategies based on the feedback from clients that have helped them to stay consistent.

1. Employ a professional or sign up for a fitness camp, this has the highest level of accountability and is my number one choice on how to stay consistent with your training and nutrition over a long period of time. There is no getting out of this one, you will need to show up and complete your workouts.

2. Buddy up with a training partner. Having a training partner can provide youwith a great source of accountability and motivation; this is far more effective than having only your self to answer to. You can't just not turn up and leave your buddy to workout on their own, that would just be plain wrong!

3. Schedule your workouts into your diary as a priority as if it was with a personal trainer; once they are in your diary your golden rule is you can't replace them with anything else. Therefore you have to plan the rest of your day around this. If you have to cancel your workout for whatever reason donate a fee to charity or have some other forfeit, which hurts your pocket.

4. Keep regular workout times each day, week and month. Training at regular times helps form a systematic behaviour, for example if you workout before you go to work, your body will begin to adapt to the pattern. It will become the norm to get up, workout and then go to work.

5. Learn some short workouts because without a doubt, time is going to be a huge factor in why you will miss some of your scheduled workouts. To combat this, it's always helpful to know a few 10 to 20 minute workouts so you can still get a workout in and not use time as an excuse not to do it. You don't need long workouts to get results; the truth is that short intense workouts will get you better results than long light workouts. If you have ever had a workout with intensity you will know that 20 minutes is freaking hard work.

If you would like to view some effective short workouts you can go to my website: www.bodyfitnesspt.com/thefitformulaworkouts

6. It's a series of short sprints, not a marathon

Two types of fitness programs to familiarise yourself with are:
1. Peaking or Development Programs
2. Maintenance Programs

You can't train hard all the time, your body needs recovery periods. A great way to keep fitness a part of your life is to use an undulating approach. It basically means alternating periods of hard work with less hard work; so if you plan a block of more intense training and higher levels of discipline with your diet, followed by a period of being less strict and just maintaining your new found fitness, you are setting yourself up for better long-term results.

Peaking or development programs are basically designed to get you into better shape or help you develop more fitness and/or burn more body fat. They should push you way out of your comfort zone and take a lot more discipline, but get you superior results.

Maintenance programs are where you should be most of the year, your goal here is to do what it says on the tin, maintain your results. This also acts as a great recovery period for your body and mind that will help you get ready for your next peaking program.

Peaking programs can last anywhere between 2 and 12 weeks. You should adjust your peaking programs to what you think you can handle physically, mentally and socially. If you are 'new to fitness,' start with short peaking programs, like 2 weeks followed by a 2-3 week maintenance, and repeat. If you have more experience, you can use a longer peak period, with any thing up to 12 weeks for more advanced people.

You know yourself better than anyone else, how to decide what length of time is right for you will depend on how disciplined you can be. Don't set yourself up to fail; I suggest you start with shorter peaking programs to build confidence and a series of successes before increasing the duration.

7. Take Action Today

If you take action and follow the strategies above, there is no reason why you can't develop a fitness lifestyle and all the benefits which go with it, like looking good and feeling amazing every day. Don't try to do it all at once, just try to integrate new behaviors gradually into your lifestyle and remember that there is no real end point when it comes to your health or fitness; it's a continuing cycle till the end of your time, it's a journey not a destination. It means a lifetime's worth of exercise, healthy eating and healthy lifestyle choices, so buckle up and prepare yourself mentally for the journey.

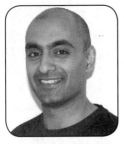

About Nicky

Nicky Sehgal has been in the fitness industry since 1999. Like his chapter, he has a successful system on coaching clients how to integrate fitness and nutrition into their lifestyle without feeling overwhelmed.

Nicky graduated with Bachelors of Science Degree in Sports Science from the University of North London. After working in a gym for a few years, he decided to start his own personal training business from his parent's garage. He now owns and runs a successful personal training studio and a fitness boot camp in Market Harborough, Leicestershire, UK.

His goal is to reach out to as many people as possible to stay fit and to live a successful and fulfilling life. If you would like to connect with Nicky to see how you can stay involved with fitness, or are new in the fitness industry and would like help to further your career, you can contact him at:
nicky@bodyfitnesspt.com
www.bodyfitnesspt.com
www.bodyfitnessbootcamps.com

CHAPTER 18

Inside the Mindset of an Athlete

By Brad Hall

Athletes are often looked at by the general public with high regard for having discipline. Not only physical discipline as far as taking care of their bodies, but mental discipline when it comes to performing everyday and under times of pressure. In the particular sport of baseball, athletes consistently have to deal with failure. Hitters who fail to get a hit seven out of ten times are considered successful. However, the success of an athlete is not always determined by his talent. Players who are regarded as having lots of talent don't advance through the minor league system because of being labeled a "head case." Players with less talent thrive and advance through the system. So how do players do it? What makes them able to handle the daily grind, the ups and downs, and the failures? The secrets to their success lie in the mental discipline that allows them to play to their potential. These same disciplines can be applied to any area of life that you wish to succeed.

Goal Setting

Alice came to a fork in the road.

"Which road do I take?" she asked.

"Where do you want to go?" responded the Cheshire cat.

"I don't know," Alice answered.

"Then," said the cat, *"it doesn't matter."*

~ Lewis Carroll, Alice in Wonderland

If we have no clear direction, how do we know where to go? Setting goals gives clear purpose and direction to where we want to end up. The more aware you are of what you want, the more likely you are to do what is necessary to get it. This helps to cut through frustration, disappointment, and fatigue.

First you want to determine what your long-term goal is. What is it you want to do? When do you want to have it accomplished? Once your long term goal is established, you must work backwards in order to determine how you want to accomplish it. This process is essential to the success of your goal. Get as specific as you can and work the process all the way back to today. For example, if I have a player whose goal is be an All-Star, this might be the conversation:

Me: What do you have to do to become an All-Star?

Player: Hit .320 by the All-Star Break

Me: What do you have to do to hit .320?

Player: Get better at hitting curveballs.

Me: How do you get better at hitting curveballs?

Player: Work on recognizing the pitch earlier.

Me: How can you recognize it earlier?

Player: By doing a vision training system, standing in on pitcher's bullpens, and doing curveball drills in the cage.

Me: How many times a week would you need to do these?

Player: Each one once a week.

Now this player has a plan of what he can do three times a week to begin the PROCESS of accomplishing his goal. Just like baseball players, you must rely on the process, not necessarily the outcome each day. You can control the process much easier than the outcome. Being consistent in the process usually leads to the successful result you desire.

A. Constant Reevaluation.

Goal Setting also involves being able to adjust to plans as it unfolds. In the instance above, if the player is hitting .220 with 3 weeks until the All- Star break, then he will have to modify his goal. Modification is an option. Giving up should not be. He could go a couple of different routes to modify his goal. He could set his goal of finishing the break at .250 or hit .320 for the last 4 weeks of the first half. With modification comes honesty. Make sure you know why you are adjusting. Not putting forth the effort is not a good reason to adjust. You might also have to adjust higher for goals as well. If a hitter has a goal of getting two hits every game, and gets a hit in each of his first two at bats, he shouldn't just coast the rest of the game and give at bats away. He could then shoot for getting two hits for the rest of the game.

B. Write it down

A research study at Dominican University found the following conclusion: Those who wrote their goals accomplished significantly more than those who did not write their goals. Writing down your goals also makes it seem more real. When you have something concrete that you can hold in your hands, your brain sees it as more of a reality than a thought. Taking the time to write out your goals also puts more time into it. The more time you spend on a project, the less likely you are to abandon it.

C. Expectations

Make sure you can differentiate your goals from other people's expectations. Goals serve you. Expectations serve other people. You can't control what other people expect from you. Once you let others expectations dictate your goal, it produces negative effects. If someone has too high expectations for you, you experience anxiety. Too low and you tend to only live up to them and not push through them. You can however use low expectations as motivation. In high school, I had people tell me I would never play college baseball or professional baseball. Everyday that I didn't want to work out or run, their words ran through my mind and pushed me to work out harder.

Fear

"Courage is not the absence of fear, but rather the judgment that something else is more important than the fear." ~ Ambrose Redmoon

Fear is one of the biggest factors for holding many people back from success. Fear blurs the line between reality and imagination. Many children grow up fearing the dark, or the monster under their bed. Only constant experiences of turning on the light proves that nothing is in fact there.

A. Bodily effects - Fear also produces physiological effects on the body. Humans are born to react to perceived threats with freeze, flight, or fight syndrome, in that order. You freeze and hope they go away, run from them, or meet them head on. With conditioning, the human body can be programmed to change the order of these reactions. Changes in the body include, breathing, tightness in the chest and muscles, heart pounding, sweaty hands, and dry mouth.

B. Overcoming - The first step to overcoming fear is to become aware of the perceived threat. Stop what you have been doing and look fear in the face. Negative self-talk is also a sign of fear. By recognizing this when it happens, you can stop it and replace the negative thoughts with positive ones. Also, by controlling your breath, you relieve anxiety in the body. Each time you confront fear, you gain courage. You soon realize that reality is not as bad as the threat. Remember, fear is the perception of something in the future, not the moment!

Thoughts
"All that we are is a result of what we have thought" ~ Buddha

One of the biggest things I hear from pitchers is that "I can't throw a changeup." Past experiences have put negative thoughts into their mind which makes them think they cannot throw a changeup. How you think determines how you play. Your thoughts can be changed, but you first have to be aware of them. Many times the wording of your thoughts determines your ability to carry them out. For instance, many pitchers when they go three balls and no strikes on a hitter, and they think "Don't walk this guy." By saying this, you once again have focused your attention on something that hasn't happened yet. You are in control of the next pitch. You have the ability to alter the course of the at bat. The mind has no ability to see the word "don't". If I tell you not to think of something, your mind will automatically see the very thing you are trying not to see. You must replace what you do not want to happen with what you want to happen. Instead of "Don't walk this guy", replace it with "I am going to come back and get this guy starting with this pitch. Throw a strike." Hearing what you want to happen increases the chances that it will happen.

A. Hoping vs. Believing
Many players go into a game hoping to hit well or pitch well. Hoping implies that you have no control over the situation, and that everything is left to chance. Hoping means you don't believe you can. As a result, you are not directing your thoughts toward success, but at a hope not to fail. You must believe that you will succeed or else the body will not put forth the effort to succeed. Belief promotes confidence which gives you a better chance for success.

B. Body Language

Many players are amazed when I can tell them exactly what they are thinking. This is usually apparent by their body language. Your body acts out your thoughts. When a pitcher stomps his foot or acts frustrated on the mound, it automatically fuels a hitter's confidence. So not only do you hurt yourself, you are helping the very opposition you are trying to beat. Body language can be changed by changing your thoughts and by changing your body language. If you are upset, and you smile for the next 20 minutes, it is very difficult to stay angry.

C. Control

One of the most important ways to direct your thought is to understand what is under your control. To obtain goals, we have to be able to focus on the things that we can control. To focus on other things is wasting time and energy. We also have to recognize that which we can control lies in the present. We cannot control the past and the future is not yet here.

We have to come to the realization that we have control over ourselves. Once we realize that certain behaviors are not out of our hands, we have taken the first step in being able to regulate our thoughts and behaviors. Mentally strong players realize that they cannot control whether they get a hit or not. As a hitter, you can do everything right, hit the ball hard and get out. It is part of the game. Pitchers cannot control what the hitter does. If you spend energy on things you can't control, it is a waste of time. Focus on what you can control.

Dedication
"Real leaders are ordinary people with extraordinary determination."
~ Author Unknown

Everyone wants to do things in life, but few are dedicated to do it. You can't just want to do something. You must have the desire to work hard. Many players recognize the need for hard work, but are not motivated to put in the time and effort. You should focus on your weakness in order to achieve success. Many baseball players who are good hitters only want to hit. If they are subpar at fielding, they rarely will spend the extra time on defense to make themselves a complete player. I often tell my players that the drills they usually don't want to do are the very drills they need to be doing.

A. Preparation

The first step to being prepared is learning. You must keep an open mind, try new approaches, and don't be afraid of doing something badly in order to find out how to do something well. One of the things I pride myself on as a coach is spending hours of research everyday on drills, techniques, and things being taught for baseball players. You must never be satisfied by your knowledge, skill, or performance. Always have a curious attitude and ask how you can apply what you have learned. If I go to a conference or seminar and take away two things that are going to help me, it has been worth it.

B. Persistence

Many times with players, they get frustrated if they can't learn something right away. Our society is much the same way in the fact that we want everything done now. If players can work through the frustration of learning something new, the end result is worth it. Many times the body goes into shock when trying to perform a new action. It takes repetitions to develop new movements that they can perform without thinking about it. The players that are the most persistent reap the rewards of getting to the next level.

C. Responsibility

Responsibility begins with being able to acknowledge who we are and what we want to become. Do you own up to your actions? How well you hold yourself accountable is a major factor in determining your chances of success. Excuses are an absence of responsibility. One proverb says, "Don't do what you will have to find an excuse for." Don't make excuses. Correct it.

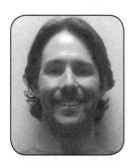

About Brad

Brad Hall, CSCS, has 6 years of professional baseball playing experience, along with 6 years of minor league coaching experience, most recently with the Washington Nationals. He has helped coach three different national teams, including Czech Republic, New Zealand, and Sweden. Brad also has been a AAA strength and conditioning coach for the Syracuse Chiefs.

Brad is currently the owner and sports director of Geaux Play Sports Training and Fitness in Birmingham, Alabama.

More information can be found at: www.geauxplayalabama.com.

CHAPTER 19

Realism For Fitness

By Dustin Williams

A client came to me one day after hitting rock bottom in her life. She had gained weight from two childbirths, couldn't manage to maintain a workout routine, was feeling unattractive for her husband, and was on the brink of an emotional breakdown. Although I couldn't relate to her on a number of the issues going on in her life, I was able to share in the frustrations of being overweight and feeling out of control of my body. I told her my struggles with weight after going through college and joining the corporate world and how a breakup with a girlfriend had kicked me back into the love of fitness. From personal experience and continued stories of similar women and men coming to me, I was able to guide her through the beginning mental and emotional steps of succeeding towards her lifestyle change.

For many people, the thought of transforming your life into a lifestyle of health and happiness seems overwhelming and taking those first steps seems impossible. Once you have decided a change is necessary, you may find yourself hitting a roadblock for the next step. The advice I gave to my emotionally and physically disgruntled client will be the same advice for you as a reader. It will help you begin your journey, maintain a positive outlook during times of high stress, and boost your self-esteem as you learn to master positive comparison.

Create Goals

Taking the first step towards a 'new you' requires not only the mind-set of dedication, but a plan of action to make sure you realistically set yourself up for success. Sitting down beforehand and creating a list of goals can help you get started towards the end results you would like to see. Whether you want to be lean, increase your endurance, or pack on muscle weight, a game plan is necessary from day one.

An important component in the creation of a goal is reality. Take a look at your current lifestyle, the resources you have around you, and the current quality of health you hold. Perhaps you have struggled with high blood pressure medications or the doctors have warned you about the dangers of your cholesterol numbers crawling upwards on the scale. Throughout my family history, diabetes and hypertension have caused drastic problems in the health of my loved ones. As I have grown older, I've seen my grandfather have three open-heart surgeries and witnessed my uncle's gradual loss of vision from diabetes. With this knowledge, I've been able to prepare my mind and body to overcome those obstacles in life and rearrange my goals to reject the health issues that have plagued my family. Realizing the chaos of your own current lifestyle and how you can change the surrounding variables are vital in the goal-creating process. If you take the time to write down these issues that surround your lifestyle, you will be more apt to take the steps in improving these areas of your life.

In addition to recognizing the issues with your health and lifestyle, pinpoint the areas of significance and discover what matters to you in your transformation. Many times, people change because they'd like to take a more active role in their children's lives, they would like to win the admiration of the opposite sex, or release themselves from the health advisories doctors impose. Although it is helpful to be specific in the goal process, such as having a weight of 120 pounds or decreasing your waist size by 4 inches, it is more important to recognize areas of your life that will be impacted throughout your transformation. During times of setbacks or high stress, leaning against those surroundings areas, not just the numbers your scale or tape measure reflects, will provide you encouragement as you go through your goals. If you have a rough week of sticking to your diet plan and your scale goes up by two pounds, having the ability to keep up with your running toddler, a task you may have not been able to do before, will be more significant than the numbers you have gained.

Once you have established a plan of action, the task of completing it is ahead of you. Keeping reality in mind, ask yourself what is step one?

What type of diet do you need to get to your goal? How many times do you need to workout per week? Do you need to hire a personal trainer? By confronting yourself with these questions, you're taking the first step in reaching your goal. From the list you previously developed of health issues and the environment you currently live in, sift out the questions that individualize your personal workout routine and diet plan. If you're a diabetic, you should be aware of the foods you can or cannot have; therefore, your diet plan will be different, as you have to maintain your insulin levels as you are exercising. If you happen to be vegan, your plan needs to include a vast variety of proteins as you workout, but it will be a different diet plan to another person who chooses to eat animal products. By forcing yourself into the mindset that you must answer these questions for success, you will move into the next stage of your new life.

After you have done the footwork in the creation of your goals, you may find it wearisome to look at it knowing all of the cardio, weight lifting, sweating, and dieting that is to come. However, do not let yourself down at this point. You are in control of your own lifestyle, happiness, and health. To lay out the foundation of your new life will be futile if you do not attempt to carry out the plan. Most people can identify the areas of their body and life they'd like to improve, but they usually lack the motivation to stick to their plan. Grab a friend, an iPod, your child, your dog, a new workout outfit, or whatever it may be to help get you motivated and go get started!

The Dangers of Using Negativity in Dieting

The groans and whines of dieters can be heard all over society. Walking in the mall, going to the gym, shopping at the supermarket, or at the local diner, the timeless "I'm on a diet" accompanied by a throaty moan can be heard. The stigma that is attached to dieting is not a reputation anyone would like to have: awful, inconvenient, unsatisfying, time consuming, costly, and many times unsuccessful. From the moment a person can grasp the concept of a diet, they are surrounded by diets that their moms, aunts, dads, cousins, best friends, or celebrity icons promote. From the grapefruit diet, no carbohydrate diet, extreme low calorie diet, to the HCG diet, the list of diets to choose from is exhausting. However, what is more exhausting than choosing a diet is battling the inner desire to repel all diets because of the shame and struggle that comes with the limitations.

Much like transforming your outer appearance, the transformation during this time of your life needs to also occur within your mind. Attaching the negativity that comes with dieting will only create havoc within the game plan you've set up for yourself. Remind yourself as you're going through your dieting and exercise routine, that you've created success for yourself through these steps. This process of reprogramming your mind to function on positivity requires continual regrouping back to your goals to keep the motivation level up. Once you can start associating dieting and exercising with the positivity it will bring to your life, such as the pleasure of losing fat, gaining muscle, a physique appealing to the opposite sex, or winning your competition, you will find more pleasure in the world of fitness.

You Can't Create the Perfect Meal Plan

The world would be a much simpler place if you could pull up to your local fast food restaurant, glance at the menu to the area your diet is found, and place a quick order of High Protein Punch and Lean Lentil Lunch. However, the world of fast food has not evolved as fast as the fitness world would like it to, and your diet is not going to be as convenient as you'd like it to be. You're going to face challenges and obstacles as you face your days of clean eating, but keep in mind the importance of changing your lifestyle rather than jumping on a 12 week binge on fruits and veggies only to jump into a bread bowl on week 13. You've already recognized the need for an individualized diet; our bodies are all wired differently, so the metabolism of one person will not necessarily support a diet another person has flourished on. With this being understood, it's also vital for you to understand that you cannot create the perfect meal plan.

Frequently, people come into my gym and they've tried the fad diets, they've lost weight, they've gained weight, and they cannot figure out why they cannot keep the weight off. With one simple question, I'm able to understand what the underlying issue is: "Have you made a lifestyle change?" A stint of a couple weeks on a diet is not a lifestyle change, it is simply a quick fix that ultimately sends your body into confusion as you plunge it back into your previous lifestyle of unhealthy eating. With the endless resources provided today- your doctor, the internet, television, the library, your trainer- you should be able to gain enough knowledge on eating healthy without limiting yourself to the point of exhaustion or to the point of relapse, which frequently occurs on these types of diets.

To keep yourself focused and not get overwhelmed with the numbers and figures, keep your diet simple. Simplicity will help make your diet easier to follow and allow you to make detours during times when you may not be able to 'scarf down' the healthy foods you had planned. The most helpful tip I can provide you with for success in your new diet is doing your research to become knowledgeable in what foods will boost your metabolism, what foods will complement each other well in building muscle mass, and what foods are healthy additions to your everyday life no matter what diet you are on. Using the resources that are available to you will only provide you with more motivation to reach your goal.

Don't Set Yourself Up for Disappointment

Most people that come into my gym can reminisce about the days when they were in high school and wearing a size two in pants, but they come in with the realistic goal of fat loss or muscle gain. Being able to identity a safe and manageable goal in your weight will also be a reflection of the happiness and satisfaction you will receive once you complete that goal. By creating an impractical idea of what you would like yourself to look like after a month or six weeks or by next year, you're automatically setting yourself up for failure and relapse when you are unable to reach that goal.

When you decide to lose fat and get your life on the right track, you usually make this over a short period of time. Whilst doing so, you forget that it took months or even a matter of years to put the weight on. Even though you may begin to see changes over a short period of time, the dramatic recreation of yourself could take just as long as it did to put on that weight. By revisiting the goals and significant areas of your life previously discussed, you will be able to make your way through those times of stress and relapse as you receive encouragement from how far you've managed to come.

Following the common denominator of the lifestyle change, it's important to realize that fat loss and having an amazing physique is a commitment. The best guys in the industry have taken the time to figure out how to stay consistent in the long haul. By being realistic on the fat loss possible and the sacrifices you're willing to take, you will be able to set yourself up for success in a long-term setting.

Birds of a Feather Flock Together

Growing up in a tight-knit family, I have always found pleasure in the Sunday afternoons spent at my grandmother's house. Even now, thinking about her homemade foods, all fried and packed with calories, makes my mouth water. We would spend hours surrounding the table, exchanging memories and stories of the week, while soaking up the good food she had worked hard to prepare. Even though these special family moments were significant in my childhood and teen years, I knew I had to make a change to make it to my goals.

After explaining to my family that I would be making some sacrifices and developing a healthier way of living, my family was supportive and not offended when I chose to find interventions while with them. Instead of filling up on my grandmother's unhealthy foods, I'd have a small healthy meal beforehand and go to her house afterwards for the socialization. Even though this wasn't the most convenient- or enjoyable- option, it helped keep me on track with my fat loss goals. Because I had also voiced my goals and plan to my family, they kept me accountable and supported me when I had moments of weakness.

Much like my experience with my family, you have people in your life that you can identify as destructive to your fat loss goals. Whether it is family or friends, you must voice your new lifestyle change to them and request their support as you will hit challenges along the way. If you have found yourself in a lifestyle rut of drinking late with your friends, sleeping in until noon, and missing the first few meals of the day, you're setting yourself up for failure from the beginning. By bringing your friends and family on board, you're able to create a motivational army to help you towards those goals rather than hinder you. Instead of staying out late with the guys every night, start with limiting yourself to two nights a week while encouraging a less unhealthy activity for the remaining nights of the week. Your lifestyle and the encouragement you receive from your peers will be an integral component of your fitness journey.

With your outer appearance changing, your diet fulfilling your nutritional needs, and toxins being worked out of your body, you will find your mind will become clearer to realize the negativity that you have surrounded yourself within certain friends or family members. By surrounding yourself with like-minded people, people wishing to succeed in their goals and become healthier individuals, you will feel empowered and encouraged to continue on.

There is more to fitness than genetics

Whenever I made the decision to start exercising and get healthy, I walked into my local gym and was immediately intimidated by high school students lifting much more than I could at that time. Although I felt embarrassed and overwhelmed to begin with, I comforted myself with the simple truth that everyone has a starting point. Not everyone could walk into the gym and bench 300 pounds; only with dedication and a plan of action could someone train to get to that point.

When you see a guy who has a ripped physique, it's not productive to think to yourself "I've not been blessed with those genetics" or "I'll never look that great!" Quick-fired thoughts like that cause you to forget the sacrifices that he's made and the consistency he's kept in his schedule. Instead of turning the situation into a negative and hindering yourself in your workout, use that image of the physique you'd like to have as motivation. Comparisons can cause you to step up your game and get out of your comfort zone.

Your perception of yourself is the key element in how much you can or can't compare yourself to others. If you find yourself judging your body by comparing it to those around you, you will be neglecting the goals and significant areas of your changing life. For instance, you may not have the physique of the woman that has been training for three more months than you, but you have been taken off your of high cholesterol medication. Keeping your mind set on these "bigger picture goals" will continue to help you throughout your journey.

The journey you will go on as you reach your goals will be a time of inner and outer transformation. By keeping your mind focused on the positivity that will be introduced into your life, you will be able to climb over the obstacles that will impede your journey. The knowledge you will gain during this time will be vital to the success of your fitness program and having those other key elements, such as like-minded social groups and a simple meal plan, will keep you focused. My client that came to me with so much negativity and overwhelming issues used this simple format to build herself up into a strong individual; she not only gained muscle mass and admiration of her peers, but she gained a mind full of confidence, endurance, and the ability to look at her progress and feel accomplished. Just like this client, following this setup will provide you with the tools to excel in your fitness journey.

About Dustin

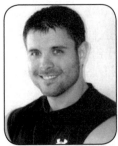

Dustin Williams is the Owner and Head Personal Trainer for Precision Fitness. He has been involved in the fitness world for over eleven years. He began training prior to going to Northeastern State University, where he received a Bachelor's Degree in Finance. After he graduated and began work in the corporate setting, Dustin lost focus on health and wellness – which in turn caused him to gain 40+ pounds. He realized he not only needed to change his habits, but that he also couldn't imagine not helping others to do the same. He went back to school and received both his IBFA certification and is an NSCA Certified Strength & Conditioning Specialist. Now he has lost 50 pounds and continues to focus on his nutritional education and knowledge. He has attended one of the most prestigious boot camp training sessions in Las Vegas, and has also trained with 4 X Mr. Olympia, Jay Cutler. Dustin has currently been training clients full-time for over 5 years, and has helped many lose weight, gain muscle, and achieve their goals. People know Dustin as a focused individual and that he is someone who will help them achieve their goals… no matter what it takes. In addition to personal training, Dustin also currently is the Regional Head Judge for Natural Bodybuilding competitions.

Precision Fitness is North West Arkansas's Premier Fitness Boot Camp for men AND women of all walks of life and delivers the best Personal Training in the area! It serves to help Bentonville residents look and feel better than ever with 30-Minute EXPRESS group metabolic workouts for busy men AND women! Precision Fitness is also a member of the Fitness Revolution Franchise.

To Connect with Dustin:
(479) 273-5707
Facebook.com/dustin.k.williams
Facebook.com/precisionfitnessnwa
http://www.PrecisionFitnessNWA.com

CHAPTER 20

Igniting Shift To Solutions: 30 Minutes For 30 Days!

By Ron Jones

"Beauty of style and harmony and grace and good rhythm
depend on simplicity." ~ Plato

Movement. It creates heat and defines life itself. Basic movement is good and accessible for all—no money or advanced social status required. Movement—life, hope, future—it's that simple.

In an age of endless exercise programs, equipment, protocols, fitness gimmicks, guerilla marketing, and opinions—most people are still not moving enough to make a health difference in their lives. Stop moving—start dying! Start moving—give yourself a fighting chance through fitness. I have a great option—for some, a real solution after decades of frustration. Got 30 days? If you are ready to leave excuses and failures behind for 30 days, this plan can be life changing for you—and hopefully for others in your life as well.

I've exercised over 1600 days in a row for at least 30 minutes per day. It's the only thing in life I have ever done with a 100% success rate—the ONLY thing. Most of the time I did not want to exercise, yet ALL of the time I was glad that I did. My daily exercise routine has a radically different approach. Allow me to share my "Fit Formula" for exercise success, because I believe YOU can learn to exercise at least 5-6 days per week for the rest of your life. Here's my story…

"Just Move!" ~ Jack LaLanne

Health and fitness is my life. I have dedicated my career to helping others be healthy. Be careful what you ask for! After my first two years as a Corporate Wellcoach, I had nearly worked myself into the hospital from fatigue. I had sacrificed my own health for everyone else's health. For a guy that believes Emerson was right when he wrote, "health is the first wealth," I was near bankruptcy.

Ignite the Fighting Spirit!

I started thinking about what I did to build my successful education, professional career, athletic resume, and many of the best times in my life—I was fit, and the best of times were built around fitness activities. Years ago, I exercised every day year round with only one to two weeks off per year. Now? I was doing good to get three or four workouts in a week. It was time for change—back to the basics—fitness first! But where to begin? I had raced internationally. I had course records, honors, and a reputation. I decided to go back to the basics...just move. That is all. Humbling, but it was that simple—and where I needed to begin.

Mind Games

"Where your focus goes, everything else follows."
~ Terry Orlick, Olympic Psychologist

Behavioral Psychology studies have shown it takes about 21 days to form a new habit, and about six months to make a permanent behavior change. I started thinking about how I needed a "kick-start" to change my behavior from only exercising a few times per week to exercising daily again.

While it sounds easy to say I'll just exercise everyday then do it, without some sort of outline or process, it probably won't happen. I coach people to exercise...I know the tricks and psychology, but now I was talking about MY OWN exercise behavior! I needed a shock to my system without adding negative stress...a challenge without crushing what was left of my spirit. I like to over prepare, so why not go from 21 to 30 days? Sounds like a nice even number. One month sounded more significant than 21 "days." From here, the 30X30 NO EXCUSES Challenge and The Lean Berets were born...and I changed my life and returned to fitness along with helping many others along the journey. I'm going to show you how to change your life through fitness in just 30 days. In an age of epidemic obesity, we need daily exercise more than ever. Let's "role."

The Set Up

Disclaimer—I'm about to make some radically different statements that oppose nearly everyone in the health and fitness business! Throw the complexities out the window with the fancy exercise equipment for the next 30 days. You don't need them nor are they important. I couldn't care less about how many calories you're burning per minute for the next 30 days. It doesn't matter! What about all those magazine articles and infomercials giving you the magic solution for a fee or that involves specialized protocols? They are flawed! Why? They focus on the body—not the mind. Get your brain in gear then your body will follow!

Igniting Shift to Solution!

Here's the paradigm shift that radically opposes conventional "wisdom" in health and fitness—your exercise intensity and program design don't have anything to do with you creating a physically active lifestyle the first 30 days, because even though my plan is "disguised" as an exercise challenge—it really is not about the body. Rather, it's about prioritizing your mind through your body in motion. Here's my plan. It's changed my life and the lives of many others taking us from not exercising or barely exercising to exercising most if not all days of the week, year after year. Ready to shift? Let's MOVE!

The Lean Berets 30 X 30 NO EXCUSES Challenge!

The Plan: There are only five rules of engagement in this Fit Formula for success. Five very simple rules that will challenge your mind through your body. It can change your life for the better—mentally, physically, and even spiritually. Prerequisite? Dedicate then execute after you declare NO EXCUSES for yourself. Interested? Report for duty below then get started!

RULES OF ENGAGEMENT
1. 30 Minutes Per Day Minimum
2. 30 Consecutive Days in a Row
3. NO EXCUSES!
4. NO Minimum Pace Required—JUST MOVE!
5. Must Be "Dedicated Time" for Exercise

"I can't speak for others, but what makes the daily 30 work for me is the 'no excuse' concept. Don't be a sissy — just do SOMETHING every day. It is like a zero tolerance policy for fitness BS. No excuses eliminates a lot of rationalizations."
~ Daniel Wolfe, Indiana

30 MINUTES: The absolute minimum adults should be exercising per day. Do it all at once or in smaller increments. It doesn't matter...JUST GET IT DONE!

30 DAYS: It takes 21 days to begin forming a new behavior and six months to create a permanent behavior change. One full month of regular exercise can truly set your behaviors into ACTION. Since there is no minimum requirement on pace or intensity, needing a "day off" is complete BS—you don't need a day off after a casual 30-minute walk, so keep going for 30 days!

NO EXCUSES: There are thousands of great workouts and types of fitness equipment; most people don't use any of them on a regular basis. STOP making excuses! If you don't exercise, you lose by gaining weight, losing mobility, and decreasing your health independence. SO MOVE! You might fight, cuss, kick, and scream until about 21 days then moving daily will just become part of YOUR regular daily behaviors. NO Excuses! Kick yourself in the butt—make it happen! You can thank The Lean Berets later...but for now, GET MOVING whether you "currently" like it or not!

PACE REQUIREMENT: NONE! JUST MOVE! Forget about sets, reps, elevated target heart rate zones, and other physio specifics for now. Mental is more important than physical at this point in the battle. Just get used to exercising daily then major "physical gains" will happen later. Keep it simple. You can always make exercise harder and more complicated, but in the first 30 days, the ***complications are counterproductive.***

DEDICATION: I've heard the "excuses" about how yard work and housework are great "exercise," yet I've never heard anyone say they lost significant weight from pulling weeds or vacuuming! When you DEDICATE time for EXERCISE ONLY, it's a *higher level of "mental" commitment.* You force yourself to step up, reach for a higher goal, and take away your own excuses. Trust me—dedicating 30 minutes a day for 30 days in a row will yield results. If you break a leg, do arm lifts! But find something you can do dedicated to movement! 30 days…NO Excuses—for a STRONGER and HEALTHIER YOU!

More Support—Exercise Psychology Strategies

The five Rules of Engagement can be enough for many people to kick-start a lifetime of daily exercise. But for some, they need a little more support. Here are some extra tips if you don't think you can do it on your own—strategies I used when I started the very first 30 X 30 Challenge years ago.

Public Support: Use "public declaration" to create more energy for your success. By making a declaration to others that you WILL succeed, it's really hard to quit. It's okay to lean on your friends, family, or co-workers to begin the 30 X 30 Challenge. When I started the challenge, I told my friends, family, clients, and posted on my website and blog. To be honest, there were many times that first two weeks when I would have quit if it were not for my promise to others that I would exercise for 30 minutes for 30 days. It's okay to get help—you will also inspire others through your sharing.

Self-Efficacy: Believe you can be physically active for life. It will happen. *Self-efficacy is the confidence of one's ability to perform a task.* The reason the 30X30 Challenge does not have a minimum pace requirement or other exercise complications is that those would decrease self-efficacy for most people just starting to exercise. ***Which are you more confident about performing for 30 days?*** Just moving 30 minutes per day, even if only walking at a slow pace or performing four aerobic exercise sessions per week at 65% or higher of your heart rate range, two strength-training sessions of 8-10 different exercises for all major muscle groups using 2-3 sets of 12-15 reps per set, plus one flexibility/mobility session per week doing yoga, static stretching, or other dynamic joint mobility protocols? Get the point? Given a choice to rank your exercise success confidence (self-efficacy) for "just moving" versus the more complex and "scientifically-validated" protocols above, I'd bet a truck load of organic carrots that nearly everyone would be more confident in just moving the first 30 days of exercising daily—NO pace required! Remember, most adults don't even come close to hitting all the official recommendations. Making your start up too complex or too hard in the beginning will be too threatening. It's not about the "exercise" in the beginning, even though this is an exercise challenge! It's about moving your mind to create a paradigm shift…yes…daily exercise instead of sedentary behaviors leading us to the abyss of healthcare disaster is quite a change. Enhanced health through movement—get some!

Moving Beyond 30 Days… Let's "ROLE"

Children and Family: We have a severe child obesity crisis—epidemic in proportions. The best way to prevent child obesity is by adults setting the example to be both physically active and healthy. It is mandatory that adults be good role models of health for children—anything less will not reverse the devastating trends which now threaten the next generation.

In addition to "adult" physical ailments that children are developing like diabetes, high blood pressure, joint problems, and more, today's children have higher levels of depression and more prescription drug issues to treat depression. There are immediate mood-enhancing benefits to physical movement! In just five minutes, you can improve mood with physical movement especially if outside in a natural environment. Give your kids a fighting chance with fitness. Teach them to appreciate health and a physical culture, and you and your family will reap decades of positive rewards instead of decades of suffering from disease and preventable healthcare costs. The start up for reversing child obesity is so simple—just get them moving because moving makes people feel better. It's how are bodies were designed to stay alive—through physical movement—not static postures and sedentary lifestyles.

Community: Once you get yourself and family moving on a daily basis, you must help inspire others in the community. The healthier we are as a society, the more everyone benefits. Health cannot be about me or about you—*health must be for ALL.* Spread the good word of health. There are no negative side effects to health! No elongated disclaimers needed for simple exercise! Inspire others, keep it simple, and help them to understand and have confidence they also can be physically active. That's the "Avenger of Health" part!

Pride and Discipline

Jack LaLanne once told me in an interview that people today have lost pride and discipline. They need to regain their pride of ownership for their own bodies! In fact, many people spend more money and time maintaining their cars than their bodies!

Daily exercise is a discipline. LaLanne admitted that he did not really like exercise—but he liked the results. It's not easy to exercise every day, but the results are worth the daily work and effort. Take action for health and fitness. Start with just 30 minutes a day for 30 days. Just move! It's that simple. Remember…after over four and a half years of exercising every single day, I don't regret a single workout. That's a 100% success rate.

While there are no guarantees in life, no matter how much we exercise or how well we eat, healthy and fit people clearly have an increased advantage for success. Regardless of what life brings, simple movement can greatly enhance your mood and ability to deal with the challenges. Give yourself a fighting chance with fitness. Make your foundation strong with health. *See you in 30 days!*

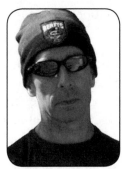

About Ron

Ron Jones has a master's degree in kinesiology with a sub-discipline in sport and exercise psychology. He is president of Ron Jones LLC in Valencia, CA and founder of TheLean-Berets.com. He is a certified Health Fitness Specialist with American College of Sports Medicine, certified RKC Kettlebell Instructor, certified Z-Health Movement Coach, credentialed Health Science/Physical Education teacher, and licensed Corporate Wellcoach.

Ron and his associates provide wellness, injury prevention, and health promotion services for corporations, organizations, and community groups. Ron has served as an endurance cycling consultant/race official nationally and internationally and presented at state and national conventions on corporate wellness and bicycle/pedestrian safety.

To learn more about Ron Jones and other simple solutions to improve health, visit: RonJones.Org or TheLeanBerets.Com.

CHAPTER 21

The Complete 30-Minute Training Session
– Feel Better, Get Stronger, and Look Like You've Always Wanted To

By Luka Hocevar

Growing up in Slovenia, I didn't want to be an astronaut, a fireman, or any other "traditional" occupation. I wanted to be an athlete.

The only problem? I wasn't the most genetically gifted kid. I was certainly less athletic than the other guys my age. But with only two TV channels to watch and nothing else to do, it didn't really matter. I was outside all the time, playing, running, and jumping.

Since then, I've always loved to train my body.

I remember lifting my first real weights at 15 years old. My mom worked two jobs, but still found time to open up a small gym. I spent hours there every day, trying to find ways to make my body bigger and stronger so I could compete. I wanted to jump higher. I wanted to run faster. I wanted to outwork the rest of the guys on my basketball team, and I knew the only way I could do it was by working smarter.

My time in the weight room paid off as my newfound athleticism got me more playing time on the court. As it happened, my basketball career took off. As the years went on, I played all over the world, from college in the US on an athletic scholarship to pro ball in the European leagues.

I even got a spot in the NBA Summer Pro League. It was truly one of the greatest times of my life.

During my basketball career, I never lost touch with training as I continued to study and become a fitness professional even when I was overseas, playing pro ball. I was hooked on training because of what it did for me and how it made me feel. Working out was not only my performance enhancement, but my stress reliever as well. (It still is.)

But while I used to spend hours in the gym, I now only spend 30 minutes. It's not because I'm lazy. Far from it, in fact. It's because over the years, I've learned more about the way the body works. You could say it was a solution to a problem.

You see, after I hung up my sneakers, I started training clients from all walks of life, most of which were very busy. Their schedules would only allow for a 30-minute training sessions with me.

Unfortunately (or fortunately in this case), I also had a big shift in life. As my training business grew, there were days when I only had short periods of time where I could get into the gym.

I had to find a way to pack everything into 30 minutes.

When you suddenly have a time constraint, you get creative. You also tend to focus on the most important things. As I reduced the amount of time my clients and I spent in the gym, I realized we were getting better results than we ever were with longer training sessions.

Nagging pains from former injuries faded. Poor posture caused by too much sitting corrected itself. But the best part? My clients lost fat and gained lean muscle, all with 30 minutes of training.

Since then, the majority of my training sessions last only half an hour. And with the results my clients and I have experienced, you couldn't pay me to train longer.

But enough about me. Let's talk about you. More importantly, let's talk about how you can follow a 30-minute training session to feel better, get stronger, lose fat, and look the way you want to look. First, let's go over the components of the 30-minute program, and why each is important.

COMPONENTS OF THE 30-MINUTE PROGRAM

1. Soft tissue quality.

Our soft tissue is made up of muscles, fascia, tendons, ligaments, and even joints. When we exercise we create "mini-trauma" to our soft tissue. This is a natural part of the training process that results in healing and getting stronger.

Unfortunately, there is also some damage that comes with it. If you've ever felt a "knot" in your muscles, you know what I'm talking about. That knot – also called a "trigger point" – makes it hard for your body to perform smoothly and efficiently. Plus, it just plain hurts.

Our goal with soft tissue work is to help relieve those knots and stretch them to help fix posture and reduce pain.

2. Mobility, activation, movement preparation (Dynamic warm up).

If your warm up consists of jumping on the bike for 5-10 minutes then doing a couple of stretches before you lift weights, then you're missing the boat on feeling better, improving your training sessions and avoiding injury.

Dynamic warm ups will prepare your body for the demands of working out. The exercises I'll show you will increase your heart rate, the amount of blood to muscles, increase your core body temperature, and help "activate" your body.

At the end of your dynamic warm-up, you'll feel loose, fresh, and ready to train hard.

3. Power/Strength.

Both power and strength are extremely important, even when you want to lose fat or feel better. It's not just for weight lifters or bodybuilders.

Getting stronger will not only help improve your muscle mass and correct body posture, it will also increase performance and the rate of fat loss. And power movements, when done correctly, will help you stay nimble, alert, and well, powerful.

4. Metabolic Training.

This type of training works all our "energy systems" and really revs up the metabolism. You can think of it as a more effective form of cardio training. It's often more intense, but since the sessions are very short, it's easy enough to work hard without running yourself into the ground.

With metabolic training, we're challenging our muscles (unlike traditional cardio where we lose muscle mass), having fun (no boring or repetitive stuff) and getting more results in less time. Not bad, huh?

Putting It All Together

While it may seem like a lot of stuff to squeeze into a 30-minute training session, trust me when I say that not only can it be done, but that it will lead to some of the best results of your life.

It's important to know that throughout the whole training session, there are very few rest breaks (or they are very short), which will make your workout more effective by creating a metabolic effect that will help burn more fat during and after the training. (It also saves time!)

Because we don't have 10-15 minutes for our dynamic warm ups, we'll incorporate some more corrective and mobility exercises into our rest periods, making good use of the time when most people sit around and wait to do their next set. We call these drills "fillers."

Now before I outline the program, I do have one small confession: my clients usually come 5-10 minutes early to work on their soft tissue by foam rolling and static stretching. (But the 35-Minute workout isn't nearly as catchy of a title.)

THE 3-DAY — 30-MINUTE PROGRAM

Below is a 3-day a week program, which you will alternate on non-consecutive days, alternating between workout A and workout B.

For example:

Week 1
Monday – Workout A
Wednesday – Workout B
Friday – Workout A

Week 2
Monday – Workout B
Wednesday – Workout A
Friday – Workout B

Repeat

Each training session will start with the same protocol of foam rolling, stretching and dynamic warm ups, after which you will move to the Workout A or B.

• Foam roll 3-5 minutes
Quads, TFL/IT Band, Glutes/Piriformis, Lats, Pecs, Posterior Shoulder, Rhomboids/T-Spine

• Static Stretches *(picking 2-3 stretches depending on the primary need)* – 2-5 minutes
90/90 Glute Stretch, 3D Hamstring Stretch, Hip Flexor/Quad Stretch, Internal Hip Rotation stretch

• Dynamic Warm Ups – 5-7 minutes

Squat to Stand x 10, Walking Spiderman w/ Overhead Reach x 10 (5/ each side), High Knee Walk x 10 (5/side), Glute Bridges x 10, Warrior Lunge x 10 (5/side), Band Pull Apart x 20, Skips x 20 yards, High Knees x 20 yards, Seal Claps x 20
Note: It may take you a couple of training sessions to get efficient with these movements and get them into the 5-minute time frame. Until then do what you can.

WORKOUT A

• Strength/Power – 8 minutes
1A. Deadlift Variation *(Regular, Sumo, Rack Pull, Kettlebell)* 3 sets x 6 reps
1B. Explosive Push Ups w/ 3 sec. pause   3 sets x 6 reps
1C. Hip Flexor Mobilizations (Filler)   3 sets x 5 reps/ side

• Metabolic Part 1 - Strength Emphasis – 8 minutes
Density Training - Complete as many rounds as possible using a weight you can lift for a maximum of 10 reps for each exercises. The filler is an exception.
• Dumbbell Goblet Reverse Lunge   x 6 reps/side
• 1 Arm Dumbbell Row   x 6/side
• Knee To Elbow   x 12/side
• One Leg Supine Bridge w/ 3 sec. hold (Filler) x 6 reps/side

• Metabolic Part 2 –
 Movement/Energy Systems Emphasis – 7.5 minutes
Intervals - 30 seconds of work/15 seconds of rest for 10 round (5 exercises x 2 rounds through)
• Prisoner Squat Jumps
• Push Ups
• Lateral Slides
• Bodyweight Rows
• Burpees

WORKOUT B

• Strength/Power – 8 minutes
1A. Front Squat Variation (*Regular, DB Goblet, Sandbag, etc.*) 3 sets x 6 reps
1B. Chin Ups (*Bodyweight, Weighted*)   3 sets x 6 reps
1C. Wall Slides (*Filler*)   3 sets x 12 reps

• Metabolic Part 1 - Strength Emphasis – 8 minutes
Density Training - Complete as many rounds as possible using a weight you can lift for a maximum of 10 reps for each exercises. The filler is an exception.
• Single Arm Military Press   x 6 reps/side
• Dumbbell Romanian Deadlift   x 6 reps/side
• Pallof Cable Press w/ 2 sec. hold x 6 reps/side
• Rocking Ankle Mobilizations   x 10/side

• Metabolic Part 2 – Movement/Energy Systems Emphasis – 6 minutes
Intervals - 15 seconds of work/15 seconds of rest for 12 round (4 exercises x 3 rounds through)
• Jumping Lunges
• Mountain Climbers
• Squat Hold Band Rows
• Sprints

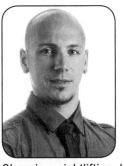

ABOUT LUKA

Luka Hocevar is a highly sought after strength coach and fitness professional in Seattle, WA. He is the owner of Hocevar Performance and Vigor Ground Functional Training Center, Seattle, as well as co-owner of Vigor Ground in Ljubljana, Slovenia.

Luka's training methods include a mixture of powerlifting, Olympic weightlifting, kettlebell training as well as many other methods to produce significant strength and performance gains, and body composition transformations. His specialty is his versatility to provide the highest quality training for every ability level – from the young athlete or fitness enthusiast to the elite/professional athletes.

Luka has trained national and world champions, Euroleague and NBA basketball players, NFL and MLB athletes, UFC and other mixed martial arts fighters, as well as athletes from multiple other sports. He devotes the same passion to all of his clients who are committed to reaching their goals – regardless of what they are striving to achieve.

His gym has been featured in Men's Health and was part of 2010 Men's Health Challenge in Slovenia. Luka has also been featured in Stack magazine and been recognized as one of the top 3 personal trainers in Western Washington.

Luka has created the unique complete 30-minute training session, which allows busy-professionals to drop body fat and get leaner than ever, but also get stronger, move better and get rid of aches and pains – all in 30 minutes/session.

To learn more about Luka Hocevar and how you can receive the free: "*Complete 30 Minute Fitness: Get Lean, Strong and Pain Free in Less Time Than It Takes to Watch Your Favorite TV Show*" videos, visit: www.VigorGroundFitness.com.

Contact:
Luka Hocevar
www.VigorGroundFitness.com
206.372.9303
luka@hocevarperformance.com

CHAPTER 22

Metabolic Resistance Training: The Fat Loss Formula

By Clint Howard, MS

Currently in the U.S. approximately one-third of the adult population is estimated to be obese... and that number is rising! Obesity is the number two preventable killer behind smoking. Health and fitness has now become a multi-billion dollar industry with more gyms and fitness centers, weight loss gadgets, products, videos, books, diets, etc... and yet, as a society we're still getting fatter and unhealthier.

As a fitness professional, these facts are alarming and force me to make sure I'm doing all I can in helping to fight "the battle of the bulge." I still get frustrated when I realize so many people don't exercise at all and many who do are going about it the totally wrong way. So often I'll hear someone say "I need to lose some weight, so I think I'll start jogging/ running." I have to tell them that just running or jogging is definitely not the most effective and efficient way to lose body fat, and they probably won't even lose much of it at all. The person looks at me as if almost in shock when I tell them this! And on the flip side of this, it's the same for the person who's been reading too many muscle magazines and thinks they'll lose weight and get lean and ripped by doing old school, slow-paced bodybuilding workouts seen in magazines. This has its flaws as well.

Why is it that so many people are still confused and uneducated on how to exercise for maximum fat loss? Well for the most part, the fitness industry has lied to us!

One of the most common workout sins I see is people performing marathon-type workouts lasting 60 minutes or longer. This includes the long, slow, boring cardio that so many people waste way too much time doing. A landmark study from the International Journal of Sports Nutrition determined that 45 minutes of steady-state aerobic training 5 days/week for 12 weeks had zero effect over dieting alone when it came to weight loss. So that's basically 45 hours of activity with absolutely no weight loss to show for it! These long, slow, drawn out workouts have diminishing returns and create a negative hormonal environment in our bodies. During these types of workouts, our bodies actually enter survival mode and release a catabolic hormone called cortisol, which causes muscle loss and results in the storage of unwanted body fat. Low-intensity cardio provides no true shock or stimulus to your body, so you acclimate very quickly and therefore fat loss results are typically very little if any at all. Back when I worked in a health club, I saw this all the time – there were members who did the same slow-paced lower intensity cardio routines week in and week out. And over the 4 years I worked there, these people's bodies never got leaner and smaller, and some got fatter while doing this.

Another type of workout sin I often see is when someone is still stuck in the 1980's bodybuilding era of working out. Hopefully most folks don't want to look like the big, muscle-bound meatheads, so why would you train like them. And of course, they're typically using lots of illegal supplements, etc. to look the way they do. An example of bodybuilding training which should be a no-no is doing single-joint isolation exercises that address only one plane of motion. Examples are leg curl and leg extension machines, calf raises, bicep curls, and triceps extensions. Single joint exercises are not as functional or practical as multi-joint exercises and don't activate nearly as much muscle, thus resulting in less muscle growth and less overall calorie burning and fat loss. Health clubs and gyms with all the fancy, useless machines are notorious for having members doing lots of unnecessary single-joint exercises on their machines.

Another bodybuilding era workout sin I often see is when someone is performing straight sets of a single exercise and having long rest periods of 2-4 minutes between sets. I'll have to admit this is one I used to do myself back before I knew any better! And you can still see this happening in pretty much any gym or health club in America... a big muscle-head dude gets on a machine or on a bench and grunts as he does a few reps then gets up and talks to his buddies for a few minutes, maybe looks at himself in the mirror for a bit or checks out some girls in the gym working out, gets a drink, then after a few minutes he's ready to start his next set. This guy may literally be in the gym for 2 hours and still didn't get much accomplished except maybe getting a little stronger. This traditional weight training has you doing one set of an exercise then hanging around for a couple minutes or so doing basically nothing productive while you're resting, then do another set, hang around, and repeat. It is obvious to see these types of workouts can take a long time to complete and aren't very efficient. Also, while your muscles are resting, your heart rate is going down so you're certainly not maximizing intensity, aerobic conditioning, and calorie burning. These types of workouts can also get very boring.

So now we know that doing monotonous long, slow, low-intensity cardio week-in and week-out isn't the best way to lose fat. And we also know that doing outdated bodybuilding type workouts with straight sets of single-joint exercises and long rest periods doesn't work well for fat loss either. So what is the most effective and efficient approach for maximizing our workouts for rapid fat loss?

Enter metabolic resistance training. The primary goal of a workout for fat loss is to burn calories, maintain or promote lean muscle mass, and create a post-workout effect so that we're still burning calories after the workout and increasing our resting metabolism.

The first part of understanding fat loss is to understand what metabolism is. Many people think they're just born with a fast or slow metabolism and blame genetics if they think theirs is slow. Metabolism or metabolic rate is the total energy expenditure of the body. Every activity that happens in the body requires some form of energy. The rate at which your body consumes energy (how many calories you burn in a day) is your metabolism. Several factors make up your overall metabolism. The one we can control and we'll focus on here is activity level, and the metabolic impact of a properly designed exercise routine which accounts for at least 20-30% of our overall metabolism. Contrary to popular belief, you're not born with a slow metabolism. If you feel your metabolism is slow, it is most likely due to your lifestyle. You are not doomed and can actually, in large part, create your own metabolism. So the goal of a fat loss workout program is to increase metabolism by maximizing calories burned while we're exercising, building or maintaining lean muscle which increases resting metabolism, and also creating a metabolic disturbance in the body – which studies show can cause your body to still be burning calories from these workouts for up to 36-48 hours later.

I'll never forget that day in my college Exercise Physiology class when our professor introduced me to the term EPOC. EPOC stands for excess post-exercise oxygen consumption and is commonly referred to as the afterburn effect. I was so fascinated by the EPOC phenomenon that I'm pretty sure it was this very day during my Exercise Physiology college curriculum that I started looking totally different at fat loss programming and workout design. And that's when I decided it was my destiny in life to be a fitness expert and help bring this whole concept to training clients.

EPOC is defined scientifically as the recovery of metabolic rate back to pre-exercise levels. It can require several minutes for light exercise and several hours or more for hard intense interval-based exercise. This metabolic afterburn is due to increased tissue turnover needed to build and repair muscle micro trauma after high-intensity training and also due to the body needing to replenish the oxygen debt that's been created.

Metabolic resistance training is scientifically proven to burn nine times more calories and fat than other types of exercise. This is due to the fact that it creates the largest metabolic disturbance, elevates EPOC, and elevates fat burning enzyme activity and total-body fat oxidation which all help to increase resting metabolism so you're burning more calories 24 hours per day.

So what exactly is a true metabolic workout? A metabolic workout features a total-body workout that employs high-intensity work periods with short rest periods in an alternating set or circuit format that combines the muscle-building benefits of resistance training with the fat-burning benefits of interval training. This maximizes metabolic disturbance creating the EPOC afterburn effect.

So what would a metabolic resistance training workout look like? There are a number ways you can set it up and lots of exercises to use. It should typically be a sequence of 4-8 exercises targeting the entire body performed in a rotating type fashion with non-competing back-to-back movements. The load or weight used should be medium to heavy resistance, the time-under-tension should typically be between 30-60 seconds, and there should be relatively short, incomplete rest periods between exercises. Generally most people don't think of combining heavy resistance training with short rest periods but this is critical in increasing calories burned and getting more total work performed while keeping the intensity high. Essentially you're accomplishing your resistance training and cardio at the same time and with much more benefits, as opposed to what most people do and separate resistance training and cardio into two separate workouts.

The high intense work periods of 30-60 seconds are glycolytic in nature meaning they burn muscle glycogen, which are the sugar stores in your muscles, at optimal rates. The more sugar you burn during your workouts the more body fat you'll burn the rest of the time when you're not working out. The heavy loading and this specific time-under-tension of 30-60 seconds is also great for maximizing lean muscle growth which increases resting metabolism. And lastly, these high-intensity work periods and time-under-tension create an optimal hormonal environment for fat loss by releasing hormones known as catecholamines (mainly adrenaline), which helps to mobilize body fat so it can be burned off for fuel.

Here is a great example of what a metabolic resistance training workout might look like:

45-15 Six Exercise Metabolic Circuit-20 total minutes: Alternate between 45 seconds of work and 15 seconds of rest for each exercise in the following 5-exercise circuit. Perform up to 4 total rounds for a 20-minute total body workout.

STATION   EXERCISE
1.   Deadlift variation (lower body hip-dominant)
2.   Pushups (upper body push variation)
3.   Squat variation (lower body knee-dominant)
4.   Rows or Pull-ups (upper body pull variation)
5.   Plank (pillar variation)

Let's look at what this workout accomplishes. In 5 minutes we can perform all 5 exercises that comprise a total-body workout. By alternating between non-competitive exercises in a circuit station format we're able to achieve maximum intensity while still allowing for a full 4-minute recovery before you repeat the same exercise. 4 total rounds takes just 20 minutes for a time-efficient, high-intensity workout which research has shown to burn more than 500 calories and elevate metabolism for up to 48 hours post-workout.

It's all about training your metabolic systems for maximum calorie burning by using high-intensity work periods with incomplete recovery. Best results will be achieved with three 30-45 minute total-body workouts per week (including proper warm-up and cool-down) spaced throughout the week to help maximize muscle growth and recovery. It's also important to change up your fitness routine and exercises every 4-6 weeks to prevent plateaus and to continue providing a new stimulus to your body while keeping you mentally and physically fresh. Combine this style of training with a sound nutrition program and there's no doubt that you will accomplish your weight loss and fitness goals!

These are the exact same type of workouts we do with our clients at my Tulsa Fitness Systems training facility and I certainly have to agree with all the research and studies on this type of training and how it compares to other workout programs. In my 12 years as a personal trainer and fitness coach I've trained over 1,800 clients and my training style and programming has definitely evolved over the past 12 years. And by far, our metabolic resistance training workouts are getting our clients the best results I've ever seen from any type of workout program. And it's also very high-energy and lots of fun, which our clients love. And I'm sure you will too! So stop wasting your time and energy on exercise programs that provide little if any results and start incorporating metabolic resistance training into your routine. You'll quickly see that this metabolic style of training is the fastest and most effective way to get in the best shape of your life!

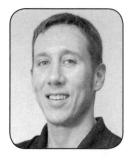

About Clint

Clint Howard, MS is the Founder/Director of Tulsa Fitness Systems located in Tulsa, Oklahoma. Clint has over 12 years experience as a fitness and fat loss expert and certified personal trainer. He's helped thousands of clients reach their fitness goals through his coaching and cutting-edge training programs.

Recognized for his no-nonsense approach to fitness and fat loss, Clint has become established as the go-to fitness expert in the Tulsa area. Clint appears regularly on the local Tulsa FOX23 News as their featured expert on health and fitness. Clint is a regular contributor for several local newspapers and magazines on fitness and nutrition-related topics and is a featured writer for the Fitness Experts Network. He also serves on the fitness department advisory board for Tulsa Community Care College.

Clint has a Bachelor's degree in Health & Exercise Science and a Master's degree in Exercise Physiology, both from the University of Oklahoma. Clint is a certified personal trainer through the National Strength & Conditioning Association and also the American College of Sports Medicine. He is also a Certified Group Training Instructor through the National Exercise & Sports Trainers Association and is a certified Golf Fitness Instructor through the world-renowned Titleist Performance Institute.

With his experience and education, Clint develops scientifically proven, cutting-edge fitness training programs at Tulsa Fitness Systems unlike anything else in the area. He delivers the highest-quality training programs in town and guarantees his clients results! In addition to the scientifically proven workouts, each client also receives ongoing fitness assessments, meal plans with quick & easy healthy recipes, monthly at-home/travel follow-along workout programs, monthly newsletters, and ongoing support, accountability, and expert coaching.

Clint's mission is to help people improve their overall health & fitness, enhance their quality of life, and build the body of their dreams. Clint and his team achieve this through professional coaching and design of exercise and conditioning, coupled with proper nutrition, in a fun, challenging and educational environment; conducive to success for each individual client. Clint upholds the highest commitment to excellence by building long-term relationships with his clients, and helping clients achieve amazing results.

CHAPTER 23

Core Concepts For Sexy Abs

By Ryan Riley, CSCS

The goal of any fitness minded individual is to have a strong, athletic body emphasized by a lean, sexy midsection.

Our quest to look better naked has generated billions of dollars in gimmicky training aids and dietary supplements that promise six-pack abs and the body of your dreams. Fitness minded people are willing to do just about anything for vanity even if it means taking some pill of 'who knows what' or doing hundreds of crunches daily, which is doing more harm than good. As a former professional athlete, I understand the importance of a powerful, strong, athletic body. Although I trained to improve my performance on the field, I also fell in love with the changes it made to my body and the way I looked in the mirror. I had a pretty good idea of how to train my body for improved performance, except when it came to training the core.

Although I was getting plenty of core stability training throughout my workout with compound movements, I still needed to spend some time isolating my core. This is where I was doing things all wrong. I was spending a good majority of time training my rectus abdominis (six-pack muscle) through variations of crunches, sit ups, and other movements that was giving me back pain, compromising my posture, and making me feel worse. I was so worried about the way I looked, that I was sacrificing how I felt and potentially performed. It wasn't until a trainer for the Tampa Rays put me on a core stability back program, that I noticed huge changes in how I felt in a short amount of time. The exercises were isometric-hold variations preventing any movement in the spine. It seemed very basic yet was challenging. I still looked the same if not better in the mirror because of the way it made me feel, which improved my ability to perform at a higher level.

As a fitness trainer, I can say that the core is generally the weakest link in the majority of us. People are getting further out of shape and spend the majority of the day sitting in compromising positions for correct posture. In addition, if people are going to train the core at all it's usually in the form of sit-ups or crunches. They do the same thing day-in and day-out, not really knowing why or how to progress to a more challenging variation. Their progression is to do more and more repetitions. This generally leads to lower back pain. I had one client mention they heard that they should strengthen their abs to prevent pain in their low back, so they did more and more crunches and the cycle went on with no results. I can't blame them for doing what they think is the best solution to obtaining the six-pack they've always wanted.

The purpose of this chapter is to provide a different perspective of how to train the mid-section not only to look better but also feel, move, and perform better. Thanks to individuals like Dr. Stuart McGill, whose books, Low Back Disorders and Ultimate Back Fitness and Performance, have strongly influenced not only this chapter, but helped revolutionize a new age style of training for core.

So, how should I train to look, feel, move, and perform better?

First, unless you have been living under a rock, you know that you can't get a six-pack by only working your abs. If you want to see your abs, your body fat would have to be low enough to show. Achieving this low percentage of body fat involves much more than the scope of this chapter but I'm going to discuss a critical component to the process: core stability. As mentioned above, the core is the weak link in the majority of us, so it's imperative that we understand what the purpose of the core really is.

I've broken down this chapter into "7 Core Stability Concepts" to feel better, move better, and look better creating a higher performing you!

Core Concept #1- Understanding core anatomy

For the sake of keeping this chapter brief and to the point, I'll quickly cover some of the major muscles that make up our "Core." The core includes all of the muscles that attach to your hips, pelvis, and lower back. A brief review of some of the primary muscle groups include:

- Abdominals *(rectus abdominis, external and internal obliques, and transverse abdominis)*
- Hip flexors
- Hip extensors
- Spine extensors
- Hip adductors and abductors

This is just a few of the many muscle groups involved, but it should give you a good idea of the complexity of the core as a unit and that it is much more than just your six-pack (aka rectus abdominis). These muscles all play different roles in stabilizing your spine and pelvis.

Core Concept #2 - The purpose of your core muscles is to provide stability for the spine.

This may sound counter intuitive but by focusing on improving the function of the core muscles that you can't see, you will be closer to obtaining the appearance you want. So by training the interior core stabilizers that I can't see, I'll be able to obtain a six-pack? Yes and no. Again, there are many more factors that determine whether or not you have a six-pack, but increased stability of the spine will allow you to perform total body exercises at a higher intensity, resulting in positive changes to your body composition and abs.

More Specifically, today's new age approach to core training emphasizes stabilization in all three planes of movement: sagittal plane (front to back and up and down), frontal plane (side to side), and transverse plane (rotational). More specifically, we want stability so that the lower back (lumbar spine) moves as little as possible when it is meeting resistive forces. The stronger and less movement you have in this area the more stable you are. Therefore, the true goal of proper core training is to teach anti-flexion, anti-extension, and anti-rotation through various static and dynamic isometric core stability exercises. For those of us that have had low back pain there's a good chance it's because of the lack of core stability. It may not stop here either; injuries to other areas of your body such as knees or shoulders could be related to an unstable core.

Core Concept #3 –
The anti-crunch and sit up revolution.

The most popular abdominal exercises (sit ups and crunches) have been the staple for anyone attempting to gain a lean and sexy midsection. But just because that's the way it's always been done doesn't mean it's what's right. These movements not only pull your spine into flexion during the act of the movement, but they can leave these muscles permanently over-developed or tight, leaving you in a constant state of flexion. This flexed position in your mid and upper back compounds postural issues created by sedentary lifestyle created by hours sitting hunched over on computers, phones, watching TV, playing video games, etc. So the question is, if our spine is already in a flexed position with the shoulders rolled forward, why would we contribute to the problem? It seems counterproductive to train your core by flexing it – which is exactly what performing crunch after crunch does. You're training your six-pack muscle (rectus abdominis) to flex your spine and pull your posture into more flexion. In addition, many studies have been done on the stress to the discs in your lower back that this flexing motion produces. This consistent wear and tear on your lower back could potentially lead to more serious issues including herniated or bulging discs.

Core Concept #4 - Train your abs with Isometric Exercises

Let's get into how to train your abs for improved performance through isometrics. An isometric contraction is a contraction of the target muscle in which tension is developed, but there is no change in the length of that target muscle (no movement). Tension can be developed by exerting force against immovable objects or by statically contracting a muscle to resist against an external force (gravity and/or added load). Your body is in a position that it must stabilize your spine and pelvis for a predetermined amount of time.

The most basic examples of static stability exercises are front, side, and back plank variations. For example, the goal with standard front plank variations is to hold your body in a straight line from your neck through your ankles while on your elbows. This is a beginner level exercise but done properly it can be challenging enough for beginners and very effective.

Core Concept #5 – Progression is key

The application of progression is critical to improved results and performance in any fitness program and training the core is no different. Progression allows for a continual increase in intensity and difficulty of exercise variation challenging the core as it adapts to the demands of exercise. More specifically, the progression of core isometrics moves from static (no movement) stability to dynamic (movement) stability.

Using a front plank as an example, let's look at progression within static stability:
A. Static 4-Point Front Plank Holds (as mentioned above).

B. Static 2 or 3-Point Plank Holds - By lifting one arm or leg off the ground you shift your center of gravity. This puts an increased and altered challenge on the core, recruiting more strength on the side that is lifted off the ground. Progressing from a 3-point hold you would perform a 2-point hold, which is performed by lifting the opposite arm and leg simultaneously.

C. Static Unstable Surface Plank Holds- Progression can be created by performing a front plank hold on an unstable surface like a medicine ball or stability ball and putting your hands or forearms on the ball while stabilizing your lower back. The ball introduces another level of progression to stability because it can move in any direction forcing your core muscles prevent the ball from rolling while stabilizing your low back.

Once you have taught your core muscles to stabilize your spine (lower back) and pelvis through the most basic static stability isometric holds, it's time to progress to *dynamic stabilization:*

During dynamic stability exercises you are challenging your core muscles to keep your spine stable while moving one or more of your limbs. Rollout variations are the most common examples of this. For example, with your knees on the floor and your elbows on an exercise ball, extend your arms while rolling the ball away from you. You should maintain a straight line from your knees to your neck throughout the entire movement. For another more advanced rollout variation, perform this movement on an ab wheel. With your knees on the floor and your hands on an ab wheel you would rollout as far as possible maintaining a straight line from your knees to your neck, focusing on zero movement in your lower back.

Core Concept #6 – Applying core stability training to your workout

Again, we all know that spot reduction doesn't work, so although core stability isometric training will help improve the function of your spine and hips you have to train the entire body if you ever want to see your abs. The largest and major muscle groups have the ability to build the most muscle, which in turn will increase your metabolism and burn more calories. With higher intensity workouts you'll be able to melt fat covering your abs.

Most of us don't realize it, but training in a functional manner through movement-based exercises like variations of lunges, squats, dead lifts, push presses, rows, presses, etc., you are really training core stability. For example, instead of performing your standard barbell bench press, try doing single arm dumbbell presses or alternating dumbbell presses. The objective is to prevent rotation in your core while pressing the dumbbell and you will immediately feel the anti-rotational stability needed in your core to prevent falling to the loaded side.

Another example would be to hold one dumbbell at your side, shoulder, or overhead in that order of progression, while performing a lunge variation. Again, your core will be challenged to stabilize an asymmetrical or unbalanced load while moving your center of gravity. This could be pretty challenging on the core even to advanced lifters who always train bilaterally, but is a more functional real world approach to training for most of us, since we are constantly dealing with asymmetrical forces being applied to our bodies in the form of carrying groceries, bags, or children.

Core Concept #7 – Quality over Quantity – The 10-second theory

The traditional thought on training isometric plank holds has been to perform an exercise for an extended amount of time. However in my experience when most people perform stability holds for 30+ seconds they end up in compensated positions due to fatigue, which limits the benefits of the exercise.

Instead, try 10-second core stability holds of maximum activation and contraction (not to max fatigue). I first heard about the 10-second isometric hold concept from world-renowned physical therapist, Gray Cook.

The concept here is to hold six 10-second max activation plank holds instead of one 60-second compromised plank. This is just one example, but should help you get the picture. You are working the same volume of time, but will get a better training effect from multiple submaximal sets than one max effort hold.

There is still a place for longer endurance-based plank holds, but I prefer shorter repetitive sets especially when adding variation and regression/ progression to isometric stability holds. Since this is still a relatively new concept, I asked international fitness pro and co-creator of Workout Muse, BJ Gaddour, to offer a free 10-second interval training sound track to help you implement this training style into your routine. (See my bio for more details on how to gain access to specific 10-second isometric plank hold workouts and integrated music to power you through your workout.)

In conclusion, this chapter offers a new and contradictory concept to the traditional method of training your core. Hopefully, you have a better understanding of the function of your abdominal muscles and their purpose of protecting your spine. Although core stability training may not sound very sexy, it will directly impact how sexy you can be. With increased stability in your spine and hips, you will be able to increase the intensity of your workouts allowing you to perform at maximal levels, which generates gains in strength and fat loss. This along with a supportive nutrition program and active lifestyle will help you achieve those sexy, lean, and toned Abs you've always wanted, and at the same time feel and move better.

For more information on the concepts discussed in this chapter and to receive free workouts, nutrition plans, 10-second isometric hold training music from *workoutmuse*, contact me.

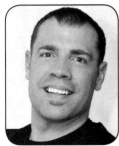

About Ryan

Ryan Riley, a.k.a. The Rock, developed his passion for fitness through his quest to become a high performing athlete. After years as a professional athlete, he started Riley Athletics in Seattle, WA. Although he began his training career primarily training athletes to become higher performing players, he's since taken the same concepts of training athletes and applied them to his programs for the general public to look, feel, move, and perform better. Ryan preaches a healthy lifestyle through sustainable life style choices, nutritional habits, and high intensity total body metabolic interval training that produce maximum results in express 30-45 minute workouts.

To learn more about how Coach Riley trains his athletes and fitness clients, or how you can receive core stability exercises and integrated training programs, or to get your free Workout Muse 10 second core stability sound track,

visit: www.rileyathletics.com
or call (206) 299-2249.

CHAPTER 24

Unstable Surface Training Myths

By Tony Rodriguez Larkin

In today's world, there are many theories, ideas, and thoughts about how to exercise properly. I'll begin by stating that I'm a firm believer in sticking to the basics in order to achieve your desired outcome (e.g., increased strength, health, performance, less body fat, etc.). This chapter won't be regarding fat loss or muscle gain *per se*, but it will shed some light on one of the most misunderstood forms of equipment found in many commercial gyms — unstable training devices.

I was lucky enough to begin my journey in fitness with a qualified strength coach at college. We focused on the basics – squatting, deadlifting, planks, etc. After several months of training, I was in the best shape of my life. My self-confidence and love for fitness grew as a result of improvements in muscle strength, muscle size, and body fat percentage.

The following summer when I had gone home, there was a shift in my training. I read some of the popular fitness magazines and started to stray from the method I was strength training in college. I started implementing exercises on unstable training equipment, which include BOSU (half-dome) balls, balance discs, stability balls, wobble boards, and low-density foam pads, which reduce or eliminate (depending on the exercise) an individual's points of contact with stable ground. I was performing some workouts akin to what you may be doing now; hops, lunges, crunches, pushups and squats on most of the aforementioned equipment. I started to neglect the more traditional strength exercises since I thought I was performing more "functional" exercises. Needless to say, I ended up losing muscle and ran my slowest times that year of intercollegiate track. Something was off.

Going into my third year of college, I had switched my major to Applied Exercise Science and started reading everything I could find to learn more about proper training and muscle function. The end of the first semester that year, I had gone from a thin 148 pounds to a lean and strong 172 pounds. I hadn't undergone any body composition measures at the time, but judging from photos, I had minimal fat gain.

How did I gain roughly 20 pounds of muscle within a 4 month period? I didn't make any big modification to my diet, except to eat a lot more than before. I had simply gone back to the basics (squats, deadlifts, etc.) and ditched the unstable equipment that I used in the past. I got a lot stronger, looked better and ran the fastest times of my life on the track that year. It was at this point when I realized that unstable surface training (UST) didn't live up to the claims.

Many proponents of UST claim that unstable devices increase perceived exertion, elicit more activity of stabilizing muscles, and enhance balance. These qualities do get trained, but is it to the same degree as its stable counterpart?

Originally, UST was utilized almost exclusively in rehabilitation programs; however, in recent years, its popularity has dramatically increased in the fitness industry. Although UST has only proven valuable with rehab in clinical settings, several companies have capitalized on this trend by marketing dozens of UST products to the general public. Additionally, you'll see a number of personal trainers misapplying unstable equipment for shock value, or as a means of improving "balance, strength and exercise intensity."

There is also substantial opposition to the utilization of UST outside of rehabilitation settings. Many believe that such training undermines specificity in programming, may lead to adverse biomechanical com-

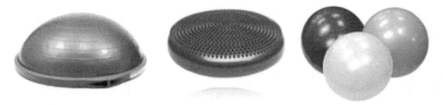

pensations, and actually impair the development of certain movement qualities. Below, I highlight some of the common myths that are associated with UST.

Myth #1: Increased Strength

Strength is defined as the ability to generate maximum external force (1). Strength training results in improvements in neuromuscular performance during the earlier weeks of training. There is a very close relationship between the increases in muscle activity as measured by electromyography (EMG) and the increases in force when starting a program. Furthermore, research done in 1981 (2), observed an increase in force production and EMG activity during the first eight weeks of training.

When the desired outcome of a training program is to increase strength, the intensity – defined as a percentage of the one repetition maximum (most amount of weight someone can lift one time) – should be high enough to elicit neuromuscular adaptations. It was concluded (3) that untrained individuals with less than one year of consistent training experience maximal strength gains, with an average training intensity of 60% of their one repetition max, while trained individuals elicited the greatest strength increases from training at an average intensity of 80% of their one repetition maximum.

The two preceding paragraphs are important to understand, because they state that strength is primarily developed neurologically at first. It's safe to say that the effectiveness of the stimulus is determined by the measured force and amount of muscle activity.

The bottom line: The stimulus to gain strength has to be large enough, at either 60 or 80% of one's one repetition max, depending if you're a beginner or veteran to strength training, respectively. This point calls safety into question. If you've utilized the instruction of a qualified professional, than a multi-joint, compound exercise performed on a stable surface can be done without harm if proper technique is utilized. I'd venture to say that attempting to use a significant load on an unstable surface for the same exercise won't elicit an optimal training adaptation (based off data I talk about in the next few pages) and is much more dangerous. For example, can you imagine someone squatting on a stability ball with a significant amount of weight? I can imagine a rolled ankle at the very least.

Myth #2: Generate More Muscle Activity

Numerous studies have shown inconclusive evidence regarding muscle activity and unstable training devices. There is evidence to suggest that exercising the core with a protocol involving unstable surfaces increases activation of core musculature, when compared to the same exercises on stable surfaces. In one study (4), the spinal stabilizer (back) muscles were most active under unstable squatting conditions, followed by the free squat and Smith squat, respectively. This study was limited in that it did not test any maximal or sub-maximal loads while squatting. Consistent with these findings, another study (5) found greater increases in EMG activity of the lower-abdominal muscles when instability was used in exercises designed to train the core (e.g., superman, side brides, plank, etc.). Note that both these studies utilized very light loads, which are not conducive to strength gain.

Despite this evidence, other studies (6, 7) found that muscle activity of the core during loaded, high-intensity, structural movements (such as basic deadlifts and squats), have shown to be significantly higher when compared to core-isolating exercises done on unstable equipment. A study in 2007 (6) found that the activity of the spinal stabilizers during both the 80% one repetition max squat (SQ) and deadlift (DL) exercises exceeded the activation levels achieved during body weight SQs, body weight DLs, and several core-isolating exercises (side bridge and superman). Another study in 2008 (7) found that muscle activity of the spinal stabilizers was significantly greater during the SQ and DL trials than the core-isolating, stability ball exercises (quadruped, hip thrust, and back extension). From this data, we can surmise that performing multi-joint, stable, dynamic exercises (e.g., SQ and DL) at an intensity equal to or greater than 50% of one's one repetition max will yield high core muscle activation.

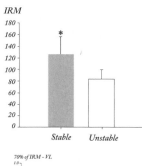

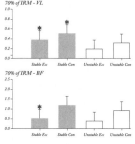

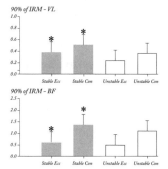

My thesis, titled "The Effect of Absolute and Relative Loading on Muscle Activity and Strength During Stable and Unstable Squatting" compared muscle activity in stable and unstable squatting conditions. We looked at relative loading and absolute loading – the first study to do so for the free-standing back squat. The relative loads were set at three different percentages (70%, 80%, and 90%) of the tested one repetition max for the stable and unstable condition. Not surprisingly, the one repetition maxes were significantly heavier in the stable condition. The absolute loads were three predetermined loads that were performed as a stable and unstable squat. In all conditions, the muscle activity within the legs was significantly higher in the stable conditions.

In my research, I found a couple studies (8, 9) that showed no change in muscle activity between stable and unstable conditions. With respect to these studies, it is apparent that the type of movement, along with the unstable apparatus, plays a role into muscle-firing patterns. Both studies had their subjects perform a barbell chest press while lying on a stability ball. The inherent degree of instability did not appear to affect the muscle activation patterns.

The bottom line: With all this data, we can surmise that performing compound lower-body exercises (e.g., squats, deadlifts and all their variations) should be done on stable ground, if the goal is increased muscle activity for strength gain. They also elicit more muscle activity within the core than most, if not all, core-isolating exercises.

Myth #3: Increase Force Output

The effect of instability and force output have not been researched nearly as much as the effects of instability on muscle activity, yet the

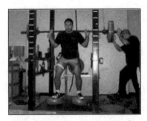

majority of the findings from the studies that are available seem to be congruous with one another. Force output is the one of the main variables measured in researching strength. In 2002 (10), researchers compared quadriceps activity through leg extensions under stable (seated in a chair) and unstable (seated on a stability ball) conditions. The investigators found that force productions under stable conditions were 70.5% greater than under unstable conditions. A study in 2004 (11) found that during a chest press maximal isometric contraction, the unstable condition resulted in 59.6% less force than the stable condition. Similarly, a study done in 2006 (12) found that when using an isometric squat, the unstable condition showed a reduced peak force output (45.6%), when compared to the stable condition. Additionally, a study in 2008 (13) established that there was a decrease in force output with a barbell chest press performed on a stability ball using the same absolute weight compared to the stable condition on a flat bench. All the results from the studies mentioned were statistically significant.

The bottom line: The primary researcher went on to state in the conclusion to his study (12): "In terms of providing a stimulus for strength gain, no discernable benefit of performing a resistance exercise in an unstable condition was observed in the current study." This statement sums up the rest of the results from the other studies nicely.

Myth #4: Gain More Balance

A study done in 2004 (14), found that a high-intensity strength training group actually outperformed the UST group on measures of static balance, possibly due to increased stabilization via enhanced intra- and inter-muscular coordination that would allow for more rapid and effective force production. Research (15, 16) has demonstrated little carryover from static to dynamic balance skills. With this in mind, one must question whether UST, which necessitates a significant amount of static balance, transfers to daily life or recreational activities, which typically are more dependent on proficiency with dynamic balance.

Another idea surrounding UST is that it will increase efficiency and effectiveness of a given exercise when the same exercise is performed on an unstable surface first. This is based on the concept that it typically feels easier to do a similar exercise on a stable surface after an unstable surface. According to Dr. Willardson (17), it's possible that the individual is actually mastering two separate motor patterns, as "the underlying neuromuscular recruitment patterns and proprioceptive feedback may be completely different" for the two exercises. Quite simply, the only way to increase efficiency and effectiveness of a given exercise is through repetition with proper technique, and instruction with progressive resistance.

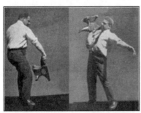 **The bottom line:** If the goal is to train instability and balance, it's far more effective to utilize destabilizing torques (e.g., unilateral training and/ or lifts performed with non-symmetrical objects as demonstrated in "Strongman" training). Research (18) has shown that unilateral shoulder and chest dumbbell presses increased activation of spinal erectors. Such destabilizing torques e.g., when pressing with one arm must be offset by action of the opposite-side limb musculature.

Conclusion

UST can be useful when performing several core-isolating or upper-body exercises in the context of a dynamic warm-up, as a component to a metabolic circuit, or in rehabilitation. It should rarely be used for lower body movements due to the increased likelihood for injury when loaded, and its ineffectiveness highlighted from the many studies above. To make the most of your limited time exercising, it's best to stick to the basic strength exercises – squats, deadlifts, presses, pulls and all their variations.

N.B. For the list of references used, graphs, and more information about structuring an effective, training program focused on instability and core strength, please visit: transformationsfitness.net and sign up for my free newsletter!

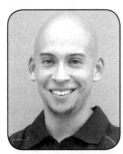

About Tony

Tony Rodriguez Larkin graduated *cum laude* at Springfield College (Springfield, MA) in the Applied Exercise Science program. He received his Master's degree at Appalachian State University (Boone, NC) in Exercise Science. Certifications include Strength and Conditioning Specialist through the National Strength and Conditioning Association and a Precision Nutrition Level I certification through the Precision Nutrition organization.

Serving greater Honolulu, *Transformations Fitness* provides businesses and busy clients the key components to maximize their time exercising. Through on-site exercise and at-home nutrition programs, Tony is able to motivate and direct the physical fitness needs of all clientele, regardless of current fitness level, toward achieving goals such as fat loss, muscle gain, better health, more range of motion and agility, less stress and injury, better sleep and focused clarity.

Tony can be reached at tony@transformationsfitness.net.

Find out more about Transformations Fitness online at http://transformationsfitness.net.

CHAPTER 25

Train Smarter Not Harder

By Steve Long

If your goal is to increase your fitness level, it is important that your workouts are intense. I think this is common knowledge amongst most people these days. In fact I've been known to deliver hardcore workouts that make people puke and/or walk funny the next day in the past and honestly enjoyed it. I enjoyed it because I knew intensity equals results.

My point today however, is not to tell people that they need to work harder. What I want to talk about today is working out SMARTER.

Making people puke and walk funny in the past made me feel like I was doing a good job, but the more I learned about proper training, the more I saw the line between intensity and stupid. The fact is, if intensity and fatigue made a good workout, then just grab a large weight, lift it overhead, and sprint up and down a huge hill for an hour. You will be tired I guarantee, but your back will hurt, your knees will hurt, and you missed out on hundreds of benefits that a proper training program could entail.

The fact is, most people's workouts are simply not effective or do more harm than good. I hate to be negative, but it's true. Honestly, one of the main reasons why I first became a personal trainer was because I was appalled by the workouts I was seeing from people in the gym. What is worse, is that hiring one of the trainers at most of the mainstream gyms might turn out to be worse than going it alone. I realized that the majority of workout DVD's were less than stellar when it came to delivering results, what if you have a question, or what if you are not ready for that level of intensity? The other options to learn about training like television shows, magazines, others at the gyms, etc., are just not the best ways to develop a fitness plan that will deliver you results.

The simple fact is that every single one of those ways to workout more often than not leaves you without the results promised, or injured. If you get anything from this chapter, get this: it doesn't matter how hard you are working out if you are working on the wrong thing or doing more harm than good.

Many people think that intensity is all that matters in a program, but now that I've been in the industry for a while and have learned more and more about the human body, how to achieve results, and proper programming, I know that not just intensity, but proper assessment of needs, needs-based programming and proper needs-based training are what get results. This chapter explains how intensity is important, but proper program design is the key to complete results.

Unfortunately, the state of the industry is pretty inconsistent. There is a lot of hype from people trying to make money, which causes a lot of misconceptions about what is right. The real fitness professionals out there know it's not about hype, it's about being smart, and finding out what is right for you.

So amidst the massive amount of information from many conflicting sources, what do you really NEED to know? Here is what I know are some important factors to consider:
I.   How Do You Know What Your Body Needs?
II. What Should A Proper Workout Consist of?
III. What Should A Proper Fitness Program Consist of?

I. What Your Body Needs

I feel that I need to take some time to explain that each person's body is different and therefore each person's body has different needs and requires different programming.

It's important to build a base to make sure that you have a solid foundation to progress from. You can't build a mansion on a shack foundation, and you can't build an athlete on a weak or dysfunctional body. Typically, people skip over or don't know anything about assessing their body and building a strong functional base with a program based on their weakest links.

This is the biggest issue that I see. People skipping steps in hopes to progress faster, but skipping steps will eventually leave you lacking on the progress you could have made, stuck at a plateau forever, or worse case scenario, injured and unable to train.

So what are the steps? Where do you begin? First thing you should do before starting any program is go through a proper movement screen and/or assessment to see what your body needs. A screen will make sure you are safe to exercise and will uncover what could potentially cause injury or increased dysfunction. I recommend finding a quality therapist or FMS Certified fitness professional to screen you to find your specific strengths and weaknesses.

Say for example that you have a significant strength imbalance in your hips, one side is stronger or more functional than the other, and you are doing box jumps in your training. With a major imbalance, repeated jumping could cause future injury; therefore you shouldn't be jumping at this time, you should be doing some corrective exercises for the hip. Instead, you unknowingly do the jumping on the bad hip and suffer an inevitable knee or back injury from the jumping, making it impossible to reach your goals while injured. Best-case scenario, you aren't getting the results you should be getting from the jumps because even though it looks right, your body is doing it wrong, and if you are doing an exercise wrong you will get the wrong results. It's not your fault, you just didn't know. Get a quality screen and you will know your weakest links and you can start to improve them one by one, until you reach the level where you can do extremely intense workouts without a risk of injury.

Sometimes it's not about giving your body more; sometimes it's about taking things away to improve results. Say for example you have some mobility issues with your shoulder. It would be counter-productive in most cases to do overhead presses until you increase shoulder mobility. So therefore, you would be giving your body what it needs by doing shoulder or thoracic spine mobility work instead of overhead pressing and only do overhead pressing when ready. Yes, you are eliminating overhead presses for a while, but you are moving forward, not backwards, with this approach. You are giving your body what it needs. Once again, without a screen you would not know you have a shoulder mobility issue to begin with.

II. A Proper Workout Is More Than Just Picking Exercises

Now that you have been screened and know your weakest links or risk factors, how do you design a workout around it? We talked about needs-based programming and this is definitely comes in to play when picking the exercises. This is the 'meat and potatoes' of your program and this is when a proper assessment really comes into play.

In my opinion, and the opinion of many other great trainers, a typical workout should consist of at least the following:

A. Tissue Quality – Sometimes fascia can get tight spots or "trigger points" that can lead to pain and/or movement compensations which can lead to a lack of performance or injury. It's important to make sure that you spend time on improving or maintaining tissue quality for over-all health and performance. Foam rolling, tennis balls, golf balls etc., are good tools for tissue work, but regular massage and manual therapy is always best. A screen will allow a fitness professional to show you the areas that are high priority, but spending some time on a foam roller is typically a good assessment tool. You feel the tight areas very quickly.

B. Corrective Exercise – This is the part of the workout where working on your weakest links is very important, and also the part when getting a screen/assessment will come in to play most. Corrective exercises are exercises that typically work on mobility and/or stability issues that you may have. An example would be that if you lack shoulder mobility this would be the best time to do exercises that increase shoulder mobility. Doing this will get you better prepared for your workout.

C. Warm-up - Most elite trainers continue to incorporate mobility and stability exercises into the warm-up also, or do not separate the two at all. If separate, these warm-up exercises are usually more dynamic than the corrective exercises to get loose, and get the blood flowing before moving into a more intense work period.

D. Power/Strength – I could write an entire chapter on just this section, but the most important things I feel I need to include is that it's imperative that you keep your workouts balanced, and make sure you are not doing exercises above your current fitness level. All of the corrective exercise in the world will not do a thing if you are doing exercises that will do more harm than good. Once again, a screen will tell you your risk factors and what you should and shouldn't be doing and where you should begin with your strength-training program.

E. Conditioning – Working the heart is always important, but make a point to mix it up with other things besides cardio machines and running. Also, running may not be a good idea if you have hip issues, or other issues such as gluteal amnesia or ankle mobility issues. Again, a screen will allow you to know which type of conditioning is right for you.

F. Cool-down/Flexibility – A cool down is needed to let the heart rate decrease after intense exercise. This is a great time for general stretching and continuing to work on your specific mobility issues.

III. A Proper Program Is More Than Just A Great Workout

A fitness program is not just a workout. A program is a planned road-map of everything that you need to take into account that will need to be addressed to reach your goals.

Things to consider when designing your fitness program should include:

A. Goals - Goal setting is one of the most important things people look over when starting out on a fitness plan. Most of the time people set some sort of goal, but in my experience most goals I've seen are usually very vague and almost never have a real action plan to achieve the goal. It's important to make sure you have long term and short term goals that are measurable and realistic. It's also important to define the true reasons why you want to achieve your goal. This is important to know for the times when it's hard to stick to your plan. Lastly, a great tip to achieve success is to think about obstacles that could keep you from reaching your goal now, and think of a few options to help you overcome those obstacles now, before they actually become an obstacle.

B. Nutrition - Regardless of your training goals, nutrition plays a huge part in your success. Building lean muscle should also be a priority re-gardless of your goals, and nutrition and training together are what will give you the results you want. Make sure that you fuel your body with quality clean foods, and make sure you fuel up after your workout to build lean muscle and help with workout recovery. It's important to make sure you have a protein shake or meal within 30 minutes of your workout to maximize the benefits of post-workout nutrition. This is a topic that you should spend time frequently researching and setting small goals each week to obtain your nutrition goals.

C. Support System – It's tough to do things alone. Make sure you align yourself with quality people and that is what you will become. If your goal is weight loss it might not be a great idea to go to lunch with the friends who don't eat healthy. Seek out successful people and you will dramatically increase your results. Find someone or a group of people to hold you accountable for reaching your goals, and help hold them accountable for theirs. It's always easier with teamwork.

In Conclusion

Now that you know what your body needs and what it takes to succeed, you can now get much better results from your workouts without killing yourself in the process. Training smart will allow you to take your training to the next level and reach your goals faster than you ever thought possible. You can't put a price on education and educating yourself about your body and mind, and giving them what they need is the best thing you can do for yourself.

I wish you the best of luck in your journey to educate yourself on your specific training needs and putting together an action plan to achieve success the smart way, not the hard way.

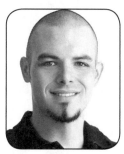

About Steve

Steve Long is the owner and program design specialist for Complete Fitness Results, and co-owner of 2 other fitness businesses. Steve has made quite a name for himself in the fitness industry by being voted Top 5 Best Personal Trainers in St. Louis in 2010, being voted on of the Top 25 Industry Rising Stars in 2011, and was also a nominee for Boot Camp Owner of The Year in 2011.

Steve has trained a variety of clients ranging from ages 6 to 80 in over 8 years in the health and fitness industry. He has assisted clients in many aspects of heath, fitness, weight loss, performance training, nutrition, and more. Steve is known for his practical approach to training and blending the many benefits of corrective exercise into highly metabolic conditioning and fat loss programs. Steve has been mentored by, and continues to learn from the best professionals in the industry, bringing the most cutting edge programs to Complete Fitness Results, other fitness trainers, and fitness enthusiasts everywhere.

CHAPTER 26

From Joe To Pro - Without Machines

By Kyle Jakobe

When I headed to my first day of freshmen orientation in high school, I thought that life was going to be easy. You see, I had grown up in a small town where I had developed a love for basketball. In no time, I was the best basketball player I knew in my area. In my eyes, this made me the best basketball player in Maryland! Obviously, my rapid ascendance couldn't be due to the fact that I lived in a small town dominated by lacrosse. More likely, my meteoric rise to greatness was due to how awesome I was. I was living the dream.

Ok. I wasn't quite this delusional, but I also wasn't prepared for what awaited me at McDonogh School in Owings Mills, MD. My untouchable mindset came to a screeching halt when I waltzed my 14 year old, 5'3", 125 lb. frame into McDonogh's freshman orientation. As I walked through the door of the athletic center, I came to the humbling realization that my head was at the same height as everyone else's belly button. My initial fear was then overcome by jubilation. I became excited that my Coach had invited soooo many NBA players to greet ME at freshmen orientation. The room was full of 6'2", 6'4", 6'6" and 6'7" physical F-R-E-A-K-S. This school is the best! I didn't know who they were, but it was pretty obvious they were pros. This is right about when everything came crashing down.

As I stood in the gym, watching the pros throw down circus dunks, rain threes from NBA range and run down the court like gazelles, I asked my coach, "Coach, who are these guys and who do they play for?." With a smile that wrapped around the back of his head, he replied, "Kyle, those are your classmates. They are incoming freshman just like you." UH-OH. My internal soundtrack went from James Brown's "I feel good" to the doom-ridden beat of Darth Vader's "Imperial March."

It was at this point I realized that I was going to have to train smarter to ever have a chance to play basketball at McDonogh. Instinctively, I had always worked hard, but now I had to make sure that I was working hard and smart. I quickly decided that I didn't like how most of the kids would walk in the weight room, bench press, talk and then leave. If I EVER wanted to play high school basketball at McDonogh, I had to be different.

I created my program based off of where I thought the other athletes' workouts seemed deficient. Instead of doing one exercise five times-a-week (i.e.-bench press, bicep curls, squats), I decided that I wanted to work a variety of muscle groups. My training education was minimal, but I couldn't justify how overtraining certain muscle groups and neglecting others was going to improve my performance and fitness level. Also, I was convinced that I had to combine resistance training with movement patterns within my workouts. My reasoning? I knew that I needed strength, but I couldn't sacrifice my ability to move. Instead of resting between sets of resistance exercises, I incorporated basketball movements: slides, jump rope, box jumps, etc. This added an element of conditioning to my workouts while helping me to hone the movements needed on the court.

Ok. So here's how things ended up for the lanky little overconfident chump from Jacksonville, MD. My freshman year didn't go as planned. I didn't make the Varsity basketball team. Actually, I didn't even make the JV basketball team! I was a starter for the Fresh/Soph boys' basketball team. Since the school didn't have uniforms for fresh/soph, we wore the reject uniforms from the JV Girls' Basketball team! Needless to say, the excess room in my chest region was a bit awkward. Life had had better moments.

Fast forward. Entering my senior year, I had yet to log a minute on Varsity basketball. After sitting out the 1st 3 weeks of the season with mono and strep throat, I worked tirelessly to restore my conditioning levels using my high intensity hybrid program. Eight games into the season I was receiving meaningful playing time for the 1st time in my varsity career. Halfway through the year, I was splitting time with our starting point guard. By the end of the season, I was still coming off of the bench, but I was logging more minutes than two of our starters. I was not a superstar. I just did exactly what I trained myself to do: Never fatigue, play great defense and knock down open shots. We three-peated as conference champions.

In case you were wondering what happened to those teammates: The starting point guard is in his 7th year in the NFL. Our shooting guard went to Penn State on a full ride for football. The starting small forward went on to play basketball professionally in Europe. Our Power Forward played 4 years of basketball in the Ivy League. Our Center still plays pro basketball in South America.

As for me? I went on to play 4 years of college basketball where I majored in Health and Physical Education. After college, I trained at colleges, high schools and gyms for nearly 5 years before opening Sweat Performance in Timonium, MD. I have trained absolutely every type of person you can imagine – 400-pound diabetics, disastrous injury histories, pro athletes, the elderly, etc. I have seen it all! Within the realm of reason, my philosophy has remained the same since high school: Training in its purest form should strengthen the body and mind while enabling safer and more efficient movement patterns. If at any point, resistance training is not properly balanced with free movement, then the training program should be altered. The majority of people work out to create a more lean and athletic physique. Well, in order to look like an athlete and feel like an athlete, you need to train like an athlete. If you want to enhance your life, boost your confidence, get in incredible shape and look like an athlete, follow these five steps!

FIVE Steps to go from Joe to Pro

1. Ditch the Machines

One of the most important parts to training like an athlete is incorporating balance and stabilization into your program. Unfortunately, most machines take away your body's natural responsibility to balance resistance through a full range of motion. Many machines lock you into a predetermined range and plane of motion causing a deep neglect of your stabilizing muscle groups. By balancing the load, machines take care of the hardest part for you! Instead of machines, incorporate dumb-bells, bands, medicine balls, stability balls and your own bodyweight. By ditching machines, you will build lean muscle tissue more easily, reduce your risk of injury, increase mobility and improve your level of body awareness. We do not have one machine at Sweat Performance. All of our clients—from boot camp members to NFL, NBA, MLL and Olympic athletes—train without the use of machines… and you should, too!

2. From Gollum to GOLLL-LLLLYYYY

Athletes, and most people in general, have adopted a train your front first mentality. This means most people go into a gym and train their chest, quads, biceps and abs while neglecting their back, glutes, ham-strings, etc. That's why many workout enthusiasts start to look like Gollum from Lord of the Rings. From both a postural and performance standpoint, placing an emphasis on the training of anterior muscle groups is very inhibiting. By strengthening the posterior of your body—hamstrings, glutes, back—you will gain results faster and safer. If that doesn't convince you, just think about how we view the body in society! In women and men alike, the most commonly critiqued areas of the body are the chest and butt. In order to make your butt look great, you must engage it in your workout. In order to make your chest appear larger, however, you need to train your back. A stronger back will pull the shoulders back into alignment and help to accentuate the chest. My rule of thumb for the upper body is a 1:2 ratio. For every chest exercise you do, make sure that you complete two back exercises. For every hip dominant exercise that you do, make sure that you complete at least one hamstring exercise.

3. Major Muscle Groups

Focus on training your major muscle groups. Do not spend time isolating your biceps, triceps, abs and calves. If you want to see serious results, you should NEVER waste your time isolating small muscle groups. By training your major muscle groups, you will burn more calories, build lean muscle far more quickly and STILL work your small muscle groups. More lean muscle results in a higher metabolism which means you will burn more calories even when you are at rest! My high school, college, and pro athletes have incredible physiques and I never have them do a bicep curl, crunch, calf-raise or tricep extension. Biceps, triceps, calves and other small muscle groups are used as secondary movers during major exercises such as pull-ups, dumbbell press and stability ball leg curls.

4. Movement in workout

Historically, working out is viewed solely as either lifting weights OR cardio. When training like an athlete, it is important to blend the two. It is not functional for an athlete—or anyone looking to be fit—to engage in stationary exercise patterns for extended periods of time. On a daily basis we walk, run, dance, climb stairs and go through many other movement patterns. Our bodies are meant to be mobile and that should be reflected within your workout. Use ladder drills, jump rope, slides, running, plyometrics and other movement-based exercises to maximize your training time, burn more calories, improve motor skills and enhance your cardiovascular system.

5. Workout with a partner

Find a workout partner! A workout partner will be your version of a teammate. They will help you work harder, stay accountable and embrace the grind of the workout. Every one of my clients works out with a group. Nothing is more motivational than competition. I know the famous saying, but unless you are Tom Brady, Michael Jordan or Wayne Gretzky, the greatest competition is not yourself! Find a workout partner TODAY.

Below, I have provided a workout that will jumpstart your mission to look and feel better immediately! I hope you are prepared to eliminate fat, build lean muscle and gain the ultimate confidence in your body. Get started now!

GYM WORKOUT

Circuit 1
A. Bulgarian Split Squat 3 x 12 each leg
B. Physioball Leg Curls 3 x 12
C. Jump Rope 3 x100

Circuit 2
D. Flat Dumbell Press 3 x 12
E. Pull-ups 3 x 12
F. Sprints 3 x 30 seconds—

Circuit 3
G. Bodyweight Rows 3 x 12--
H. Glute Bride 3 x 12
1. Slides 3 x 30 seconds

EXERCISE FORMAT

A. Bulgarian Split Squat

Stand in a stationary lunge position. Place your rear foot firmly on top of a bench or box no higher than 18 inches. Set your core and maintain an erect torso as you descend until your thigh is parallel to the ground. Keep your front heel firmly on the floor throughout the motion. You should feel a stretch in your rear leg's hip flexor as you descend. Drive upward and exhale as you ascend out of the deep lunge. Complete all repetitions with one leg, then switch to the other leg to complete the same number of reps. Start using bodyweight, but progress to holding dumbbells or using a barbell across your shoulders.

B. Physioball Leg curls

Lying flat on the ground on your back, place your legs (just below your calf) up on a Swiss ball, toes pointed up with hips on the floor. Start by pressing your hips up so that your shoulders, hips and ankles are in a straight line. Pull the ball in towards your body by flexing your knee and extending your hips into the air. In a controlled motion, let the ball back out until you are in the starting position. That is one repetition. Your knees, hips and shoulders should remain in line during all parts of the exercise.

C. Jump Rope

Using a jump rope, mix in two-foot, one-foot, side-to-side, front-to-back and double jumps. All jump rope sets should be completed by reps, not time. Otherwise you may find yourself making purposeful mistakes as your precious time slips away!

D. Flat DB Press 3 x 10

Perform a flat DB press by evenly lowering the weights down and out until your elbows drop just slightly below ninety degrees. Drive the weights up and in until your arms are fully extended. Your wrists should remain over your elbows throughout the range of motion

E. Pull-ups:

Using a neutral grip (palms facing in towards each other) with hands no wider than shoulder width, start in a complete hanging position under a fixed bar. Lifting your chest up, drive your elbows out and down to raise your body until your chin is above the bar.

F. Sprints
Using a treadmill, elliptical or open space, perform 30 seconds of high intensity cardio.

G. Bodyweight Rows
Lie on the floor underneath the bar (which should be set just above where you can reach from the ground). Grab the bar with an overhand grip (palms facing AWAY from you). Contract your abs while keeping your ears, shoulders, hips and ankles in a straight line. Pull yourself up until your chest touches the bar. Lower yourself back down.

H. Glute Bride
Lie face up on the ground with your arms to the side, knees bent, and heels on ground. Lift hips off the ground until knees, hips, and shoulders are in a straight line. Hold 2 -3 seconds, return to start position and repeat for prescribed number of repetitions

I. Slides
Using any open space, shuffle laterally for 30 seconds. During the movement, keep your chest out, shoulders back and knees bent so that you remain in a half-squat. Try placing two markers 5, 10 or 15 yards apart from one another. Slide back-and-forth between the markers as fast as possible for the prescribed period of time.

Are you interested in an athlete workout that requires no equipment at all? Check out the Press Box section of www.sweatperformance.com and look for, "The Weightless Workout!"

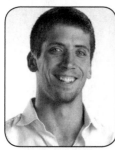

About Kyle

Kyle Jakobe is the owner of Sweat Performance—an elite sports performance facility located just north of Baltimore, MD. He has been featured as a fitness expert on Fox Sports Radio, ESPN Radio, PressBox Live Sunday and the MASN Channel. Kyle has been the strength coach at the prestigious McDonogh School in Owings Mills, MD for the past 5 years. Over that time, McDonogh has proven itself to be one of the most dominant high school sports programs in the entire eastern region.

In addition to operating the Sweat Performance business, Kyle trains athlete groups and adult boot camps within his facility. He currently trains athletes who compete at the professional, collegiate and high school levels. He has trained All-Americans, Collegiate National Player of the Year recipients, NFL Pro Bowlers and NCAA National Champions.

Kyle also runs Kobe Performance - a basketball skills-development program. Through Kobe Performance, he has produced over 30 Division 1 basketball players and 30 professional basketball players.

To learn more about Kyle Jakobe and how you can improve your performance, body and life, visit: www.sweatperformance.com

CHAPTER 27

How To Design 'Guaranteed Results' Training Programs

By Jon Le Tocq

When I first qualified as a trainer, I worked at the typical chrome-plated leisure club that looked like an Egyptian bazaar where members chose whatever took their fancy each day. The concept of following a set program that would DEFINITELY produce results, was deemed 'unnecessary' by many.

One day I approached a middle-aged guy on the 'pec dec' with a super-size spare tyre. I suggested a few changes to his program and got a reply I will never forget.

"Thanks son, but I've been doing the same program for nine years, so I don't need all your new fancy stuff."

NINE YEARS IN THE GYM AND STILL FAT!

I wish I could say this was a rare occurrence, but it's now a rarity to find someone who HAS got the body they want. I had to get out and work with people who genuinely want to see change, be the change and not just be entertained with TV's and lycra.

I'm still learning and always will be, but with more and more people qualifying as gym instructors and personal trainers, yet rapidly increasing rates of obesity and ill health, I can categorically state one thing: Most of the industry is getting it seriously wrong in attempts to just entertain or sell stuff.

Having worked with a professional rugby player, Guernsey First XV Rugby, Guernsey Cricket, numerous amateur athletes, a lady who went from 20 stone 10 to 10 stone 5, nurses, GP's, office workers, lawyers, under 18's, mums and just about every profession you can imagine, I've seen a few things work, but many more fail. The catch is that some programs can be guaranteed to work for some people, but not others.

Here's what I know so far…

Balanced Programs

Guaranteed results programs don't look at balance in terms of working opposing muscles the same — but aligning where you are now with where you want to be.

Desk Jockey Dave is a round-shouldered office worker. Performing equal numbers of sets and reps on his chest and upper back will simply make him bigger or at least stronger in the same poor position. His risk of shoulder injury or back problems will not improve and will most likely get worse unless he starts to work more on his back than on his chest to address the existing imbalance.

Desk Jockey Dave's glute muscles are also likely to be suffering from some kind of dysfunction due to sitting down all day. He thinks he is doing the right thing by doing lots of squats, deadlifts and lunges for a 'balanced' workout, but in fact he is overloading those muscles which have to compensate for glute weakness, in particular his lower back. This is made worse in the presence of poor ankle or hip mobility.

At the other end of the spectrum, focusing all your efforts correcting the posture of a rugby player or cyclist, can in fact DETRACT from their performance. In the grand scheme of life it may help these people to improve their posture, but in terms of their sport, performance may well drop because their body has adapted to an optimal position for their sport which you are now trying to break down.

What's optimal for elite sport, fast muscle gain or movie star fat loss, isn't always optimal for health and vice-versa. Whilst health should feature heavily in all programs, there is a need to switch between methods if particular goals are required…and fast.

"If all you have is a hammer, everything begins to look like a nail".

Don't try to create a program based on entertainment – you can't guarantee results that way. For instance, if you want to complete a sub 1 hour sprint triathlon, don't do 2-3 hours per week 'pumping the guns' or doing torturous 1 hour conditioning sessions.

Be specific. Every session and every exercise moves you closer to, or further away from, your goal.

Make Room For Success

Is there room in your life for the Guaranteed Results program? If it is impossible to fit it in with your responsibilities as a parent, employee or business owner, the program will fall flat.

Sacrifices need to be made to be successful in anything, but they also need to 'fit' certain other criteria.

How To Make The Program Fit

Health and fitness programming has become about how many sets and reps are required for strength versus power; endurance versus muscle growth. It seems so long as we get these right, we know we're in the ballpark for good results.

Unfortunately, these factors are sometimes the LAST piece of the jigsaw – particularly outside of the elite sport world where training and competition is often the only concern.

Take Desk Jockey Dave.

His mate has stacked on 10kg of muscle in six months, training six times each week. Dave fancies a piece of the action since seeing his muscular body disappear when the kids arrived on the scene...

He tries the program for two weeks then finds his muscles ache all the time, he's falling asleep at work and he's put on virtually no muscle.

Now, Dave and his wife have two kids to run around after on top of his stressful finance job, and his levels of the stress hormone cortisol are through the roof. Cortisol is affected by chronic stress levels and not only does it have a catabolic affect on muscle tissue, but it also creates systemic inflammation, greatly affecting recovery. The program is now just piling more stress on to Dave's body and mind and dragging him down further.

Dave's wife Caroline is also failing to see any results at her new Intense Bootcamp combined with a high protein, low fat, low carb diet, even though it did wonders for her friend. No matter how hard Caroline tries, the weight won't shift, so she cuts more calories. Now she's tired all the time and gets severe hunger cravings resulting in Saturday night binges. She's actually putting on weight!

Again, the reason is that the program is not right for CAROLINE. It works for her friend who can relax by the pool and have a sauna whilst Caroline tears her hair out running around after the kids.

Caroline is also a serial dieter. Every diet she has done has further disrupted her hormones including her insulin (controls blood sugar) and leptin (controls hunger and appetite).

In between crazy starvation diets, Caroline binges and eats lots of bad food, so her digestive system is clogged up with processed food and high levels of meat − dragging her energy levels down even more. Leptin is no longer produced properly in Caroline, so she doesn't get the proper "I'm full" signals, hence the constant hunger pangs.

Her adrenal glands are also malfunctioning, unable to keep producing high levels of adrenaline to cope with all the daily stresses and challenges. So the bootcamp which SHOULD bring fat loss doesn't work for Caroline. She doesn't have the energy to train hard, and the high protein diet isn't helping because it's dragging her energy levels down even further.

What should Caroline do?

Cardio, Weights, Aerobic Exercise or High Intensity Interval Training?

There are so many ways to train it can look like a minefield! Go on the internet and you'll see people arguing over long-steady cardio, intervals or no cardio. Some favour heavy strength training for joint and ligament health as well as muscle gain, whereas others never go near weights for fear of 'bulking up'.

The truth is that ALL of the different modes have incredible value in guaranteeing results in certain situations. The key to programming them in requires looking at the individual's goals and their current stress levels, fitness levels, time availability and body type.

For instance, metabolic conditioning with kettlebells, ropes and tyre-flipping is a fantastic way to increase work capacity, burn body fat and rapidly increase stamina levels FOR SOME PEOPLE. However, for a stressed-out office worker and single Mum of three, it may be the straw that broke the camel's back.

When an individual's 'stress bucket' starts to brim over, it can manifest itself as backache, depression, weight-gain, illness or mood swings. In this case, the best choice would be a relaxation program including some deep breathing or yoga, mind-awareness coaching and light aerobic cardio program which gets the individual out in the open air and oxygenates their blood. The emotional freedom associated with running can make an instant difference to mood and hormones, greatly improving the chances of success.

The cardio work could involve some basic bodyweight movement patterns, but in such a way that doesn't involve working to failure or stress. Lets assume Caroline can perform 10 good repetitions of bodyweight squats, push-ups and reverse lunges. A good way to start training would be performing 5 sets of 5 reps of each exercise to introduce movement and training principles without smashing her into the floor!

At first, I wouldn't even time any runs or measure distances. Just let Caroline have some fun and leave with a feeling of progress and accomplishment. Use some boxing to de-stress and get a good sweat on. Caroline should not be attempting to become the next Miss CrossFit 2011 just yet!

The Fantastic Four For Highly-Stressed People

If you are permanently stressed, you should look to optimize…

1 - Oxygenation
2 - Perspiration
3 - Defecation
4 - Urination

Ensure totally clean nutrition, controlling animal protein consumption.

Drink loads of water and schedule some light, relaxing exercise. This will help reset hormones, flush out toxins which drag energy levels down and affect brain performance, improve digestion and optimize metabolic function for fat burning.

The key to program management going forward lies in knowing when to 'up the pace', but there is no black-and-white answer. It takes careful observation.

When you see life come back and a zest for exercise reappear, you can start introducing fitness tests, and bring in some free-weight training, progressing to harder sessions. The session structure is dependent on the goal, not what you like doing!

Be prepared however, to take a step back should life become too stressful again, making it difficult to cope with hardcore training on top.

If You Can't Gain, Don't Train

You either move forwards or backwards with fitness training – there is no in-between!

The key lies in getting to know yourself and recording your physical and mental reactions to times of stress, methods of training and the results.

Track...
1) Your weight and body fat
2) Performance indices such as your favourite 5k run or weights lifted
3) Your emotions and energy levels as the program progresses
4) Your resting heart rate
5) Your blood pressure

These five factors will tell you all you need to know about whether Guaranteed Results are around the corner.

The Guaranteed Results Program

You should have realized by now that recommending one program is like playing 'Pin-The-Tail-On-The-Donkey.' Instead, here are the principles for different goals for you to grasp and apply daily.

In addition to the points below, all categories require adherence to a clean, natural diet, the details of which can't be covered sufficiently here. However, if you only drink 2-3 litres of filtered water eat lean, organic proteins, lots of vegetables, healthy fats and keep starchy carbs to post-training meals, you won't be far off!

1. STRESSED OUT BUSY BODY

You need to...

...reset hormones by making time for relaxation, breathing and an absence of technology and sources of stress.

...introduce light aerobic work, which can include bodyweight exercises and traditional cardio (taking into consideration impact and obesity factors)

...avoid stressful, anaerobic exercise for the first few weeks.

Typical session:

Movement preparation circuit	15 minutes
Boxing 5 rounds of 1 min 30 with 1 min 30 light jog to recover	
Dynamic stretching and yoga movements	10 minutes
Seated deep breathing	10 minutes

2. FAST FAT LOSS (ASSUMING LOW DAILY STRESS LEVELS)
You need...

...full body resistance sessions 3-4 times per week

...sessions beginning with hypertrophic work and ending with metabolic conditioning work (high intensity, short rest breaks and 'Timed' challenges of 10-15 minutes)

...possibly extra aerobic intervals 2-3 times per week (6-10 x 200-400m @80% of max effort on each interval with walk back or jog back recovery). This may be unnecessary if you are a tall, lean body ectomorphic body type.

Typical session:

A1: Overhead press	3 x 8 reps	30 seconds rest
A2: Reverse lunge	3 x 10 reps each side	30 seconds rest
B1: Step up	3 x 8 reps each side	30 seconds rest
B2: Push up	3 x 15 reps	30 seconds rest

Finisher:
As Many Rounds As Possible in 15 minutes...
20 burpees
100m sprint
50 reps on battling ropes

3. MUSCLE BUILDING
This is another area in which one size doesn't fit all.

A boxer may want to gain weight but maintain his lethal, lightning bolt of a right hook – so he should not be performing slow grinding bench presses which reduce his rate of force production. He also won't want to ache so much that he can't lift his arms tomorrow!

A bodybuilding competitor however, may not care how fast he can punch, and slow repetitions may work better for tearing muscle apart ready for being rebuilt bigger.

A rugby player might need more size, and so needs to be packing on muscle and gaining strength for performance.

So we might look at a strength-hypertrophy program (with the focus on hypertrophy) in the off-season, moving to a greater focus on strength and power as we get closer to the start of the next season.

In all circumstances, I would always have a Big Bang heavy strength exercise at the start of each session such as squat, deadlift or overhead press followed by non-competing supersets. I would also add some sprints for the athletes.

The method, rep ranges and tempo of lifting would change if we want to guarantee results for all three guys.

Typical upper body session:
A1: Hang clean   5 sets of 5   60 seconds rest
B1: Overhead press   7-9 reps, 3-5 reps, 10-12 reps
B2: Single arm row   10-12 reps, 6-8 reps, 12-15 reps
C1: Reverse ab curl   3 sets of 15   30 seconds rest

If you need to shed some fat, finish with 10-15 minutes intense conditioning work such as battling ropes, tyre flips and kettlebell complexes.

There is no need to over-complicate things with twelve different exercises.

Go heavy and go hard on the basics.

Guaranteed Results

The only way to 'guarantee results' is to get everything spot on for each individual's goals and current physical, emotional and lifestyle status. To do this requires awareness of what's happening day-to-day, week by week and month-on-month.

If you can't do this for yourself, hiring a trainer is essential – otherwise you face years of playing Pin-The-Tail-On-The-Donkey in the gym.

There ARE Guaranteed Results out there for you, but they don't come in a 'done- for-you' neatly packaged DVD!

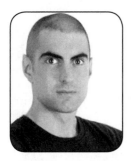

About Jon

Jon Le Tocq was voted UK Personal Trainer of the Year 2011 and owns Storm Force Fitness, Guernsey's leading body transformation company.

You know those days when you look great, have loads of energy and feel invincible?

Jon makes that happen.

He and his team of trainers help over 150 people per week achieve their body transformation and sports performance goals – through the Guernsey Fitness Camp, strength and conditioning for teams and exclusive personal training services.

Founding Storm Force Fitness in 2009, Jon has rapidly established himself as the 'no nonsense' trainer who inspires his clients and followers to achieve much more than they thought possible, with a talent for pushing the right buttons at the right time.

Having studied with some of the world's leading experts, Jon has an arsenal of training and nutrition weapons for any goal, fast-tracking his clients through their programs in record time.

Jon's fat loss and strength and conditioning expertise are highly sought after in Guernsey, with the leading sports teams training with Storm Force Fitness in order to rise up the national and international divisions, and hundreds of individuals attending his various workshops and seminars.

To learn more about Jon Le Tocq and how you can work with Storm Force Fitness in person or online, visit: www.stormforcefitness.com
or email: info@stormforcefitness.com .

CHAPTER 28

Self-Limiting Exercises

By Alwyn and Rachel Cosgrove

First introduced to the term 'self-limiting exercise' a few years ago while speaking with Gray Cook (while teaching together at a Perform Better one-day event). Gray was talking about the book Born to Run by Christopher MacDougall and the 'barefoot running' idea.

Running barefoot is what can be classified as a self-limiting exercise – the body cannot over-stride or heel strike because the immediate feedback (in this case – pain) auto-corrects the form of the runner. In fact, it is completely self-limiting as there is no way of creating overuse injuries either – the foot and the joint impacts of running will prevent overuse as you'll stop running. You can't do it incorrectly.

Barefoot running then is essentially a perfect exercise. However – when we introduced the running shoe with padding – we put a problem in there. But, to be completely fair, shoe manufacturers thought they were creating a solution. The body, when wearing padded shoes, is now no longer given immediate feedback to adjust or correct running form, and the very nature of the thick sole of the shoe can allow runners to perform far more volume than their muscles and joints can handle with poor running form. The results? Inevitable injuries, as exhibited by many, strapped up, knee-supported runners you see.

A self-limiting exercise, as defined by Gray "requires mindfulness and an awareness of movement, alignment, balance and control. In self-limiting exercise, a person cannot just pop on the headphones and run or walk on the treadmill fingering a playlist or watching the news on a well-placed monitor. Self-limiting exercise requires engagement"

Adding to this definition is that a self-limiting exercise provides an automatic, yet natural obstacle or built in "abort" mechanism that prevents you from doing the exercise wrong, or doing an excessive volume.

I suppose my first exposure to self-limiting exercise was via martial arts training, and in particular sparring – if you don't protect yourself, you get hit – immediate feedback in the form of a punch on the nose!

Another example is stair climbing. Near our house, there are about 80 stairs going up the side of a hill where many people frequently get their workout done. Stair climbing is also self-limiting. You can either pick your foot up and step up to the next step or not. You may need to slow down or if you are in great shape, you can run up the stairs. If you are not strong enough or fit enough you simply will not be able to climb the stairs and it is hard to do it wrong, you just won't be able to do it. You can either step up or not.

With speed and agility training, the CHAOS system, as devised by Robert Dos Remedios of open-response is self-limiting – athletes are left behind or fall if their technique or direction change isn't perfect – very different from closed-response (when you know when you're going to change direction).

At Results Fitness we have realized that it also applies to many of the traditional exercises we use. For example – The Turkish Get-up, inverted rows, bottoms-up kettlebell pressing are all self-limiting. It's hard to do too many bottoms-up presses; you won't be able to keep the kettlebell in position.

With inverted rows – either the core, or the grip strength limits you. And with Turkish get-ups – you'll either remain stuck to the floor or have a weight drop on your head! There are more – jump rope can't be performed incorrectly or to excess, the battling ropes system, suspension training and the stability ball all have built-in corrections or "abort" mechanisms in their very nature.

As we studied the concept of self-limiting exercise more, we started to think of it in terms of fat loss training. In fact, self-limiting exercise may be one of the reasons why our fat-loss programs at Results Fitness are so successful. Self-limiting exercise performed in a circuit is essentially training to technical failure, but without the risk of overuse injury or sloppy form – it's just impossible to do poor, sloppy reps. Yet the energy demands are through the roof. To train with that absolute level of engagement demands so much metabolically that it can be exhausting and immediate in terms of fat-loss results, yet at the same time being of a low volume due to the auto-correction mechanisms in place.

Anecdotally, did a recent workout of Turkish Get-ups. Performing a countdown style workout with 60s rest between sets: 5 reps each side, 4 reps, then 3, 2 and finally a single rep. The last rep took almost as long as the first set of five. The entire workout, including rest periods, took less than 20 minutes and consisted only of 30 total repetitions. It was mentally and physically tough however - almost exhausting. Despite being low in volume, and short – the metabolic demands were off the charts.

Can self-limiting exercise be the future of fat-limiting exercise? Naturally imposed loads seem to train the weakest links, with a high metabolic cost – naturally!

To summarize, what makes an exercise self-limiting?
• Body is given *immediate feedback* (you immediately know you when you are doing it wrong)
• Any exercise that is governed by grip strength, breathing, balance, postural alignment or co-ordination
• Hard (but not impossible) to do incorrectly
• Requires mental engagement – Gray cook calls this, "Forced Focus"
• It can be auto corrective

What *self-limiting exercises* are not....
• Automatic cure alls
• Too difficult to do (they must be appropriately challenging)
  Here are some examples of some of the self-limiting exercises that we employ regularly at Results Fitness:
• ½ and tall kneeling chops and lifts (balance and small base of support)
• ½ and tall kneeling bottoms up kettlebell presses
• Any "bottoms up" (holding the kettlebell by the handle upside down) pressing or squatting movement with kettlebells – you'll lose the positioning if the core is not tight or the grip strength isn't there
• Medicine ball throws from various stances – power is inherently self limiting

- Turkish Get-ups (this may be the best example of a self-limiting exercise that there is)
- Farmers walks (walking carrying heavy dumbbells on one side of the body) – this is self-limiting due to posture, core stability and co-ordination
- Suspension training rows and/or push-ups
- Single-leg squats
- Goblet position squats
- Any offset-loaded lower body exercises
- Using heavy ropes (battling ropes style)
- Chin-ups
- Running uphill or downhill
- Sled pushes and or drags

Here's a sample self-limiting workout.

Core

1. Planks with feet on stability ball – hold for 60s.

2. ½ kneeling cable chops – select a weight that will allow ten reps without breaking technique – Perform 2 sets each side with 30s rest between sets.

3. Suitcase walks – hold a heavy dumbbell in one hand – walk 50 yards keeping your other arm behind your back and your torso erect. Change hands and repeat.

Resistance Training

1: Turkish Get up: Perform 3 sets of 5 reps each side resting 60s between sets.

2a: Goblet Squat – select a load that allows ten reps.

2b: Push-ups with one foot on a stability ball – perform as many reps as possible.

2c: Inverted-row – as many reps as possible.

Perform as many rounds as possible in 15 mins.

3a Chin-ups – try to stop one rep short of failure.

3b: Single arm bottoms up kettlebell press (start with your weakest side – do as many reps as possible and match that on your strong side).

3c: Reverse Lunges with one heavy dumbbell held at shoulder height (same side as the front leg) – use a load that allows ten reps per side.

Perform as many rounds as possible in 15 mins.

Metabolic

Pick heavy ropes and jump rope. Alternate between the exercises for 30s on, 30s off for 10 total minutes (5 rounds of each).

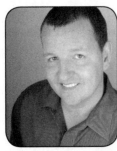

About Alwyn

Born in Scotland and initially exposed to fitness training through an intense competitive sport/martial arts background, Alwyn Cosgrove began reading and studying any training-related material he could get his hands on. This led Alwyn to formal academic studies in Sports Performance at West Lothian College and then progressed on to receiving an honors degree in Sports Science from Chester College, the University of Liverpool.

During his career as a fitness coach, Alwyn began with assisting in martial arts lessons in 1986 and teaching fitness classes in 1989. He has studied under all of the top fitness professionals and coaches in the world and has worked with a wide variety of clientele, from general population clientele to several top-level athletes.

A sought-after 'expert' for several of the country's leading publications, including a regular contributor to *Men's Health* magazine, Alwyn has co-authored three books in the "*New Rules of Lifting*" series. He currently spends his time consulting on fitness training, training clients, training his staff at Results Fitness, speaking on the fitness lecture circuit and coaching fitness trainers worldwide in their businesses.

For the past decade, with his wife Rachel, Alwyn runs Results Fitness in Santa Clarita, California - which has twice been named one of America's Top Gyms by Mens Health magazine, a gym which specializes in programs for real-world busy people, and prides itself on "changing the way fitness is done – period!"

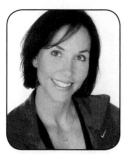

About Rachel

Rachel co-owns and operates Results Fitness with her husband Alwyn Cosgrove, a fitness center in Southern California for over 11 years. It was voted one of the top 10 gyms in the United States three years in a row by *Men's Health* Magazine. She earned her Bachelor of Science in Physiology at the University of California at Santa Barbara and holds her CSCS with the National Strength and Conditioning Association. She has also been certified by the International Society of Sports Nutrition, USA Weightlifting and with Precision Nutrition.

Rachel has been featured in numerous magazines including *Muscle and Fitness Hers, Men's Fitness, Men's Health, Women's Health, Oxygen, More Magazine, Runner's World, Women's World, Real Simple, More Magazine, Shape* magazine among others.

She currently has her own column in Women's Health Magazine and is the best selling author of the book *The Female Body Breakthrough*, published by Rodale in November 2009. She has also been interviewed on television on Fox, ABC and WGN numerous times discussing her book and sharing her message.

As one of the featured speakers for the company, Perform Better, she lectures nationally and internationally on topics such as strength training, fat loss, business in the fitness industry and nutrition, specifically for women, helping them to reach their potential in all aspects of their life.

Rachel is also an athlete herself. She is an Ironman Triathlete and has been to the World Championships on Team USA for triathlon. She has also competed in Powerlifting and fitness competitions. Extremely goal oriented, she is always looking for a new physical challenge and draws from that experience – making her a better coach.

As a spokesperson for Secret Deodorant and Nike, she has also been a consultant for Gatorade, Nike, *Women's Health* and *Men's Health* Magazines.

She and her team at Results Fitness strive to become the best part of their member's day, achieving results and changing lives while having fun doing it! They are on a mission to change the way fitness is done.

You can learn more about Rachel at: www.rachelcosgrove.com and Results Fitness at: www.results-fitness.com.